The Psychedelic Anthology is a seven-part anthology and collection of real-life psychedelic experiences shared from all over the world. This anthology challenges the negative stigma surrounding sacred medicines such as LSD, Ayahuasca, and Mescaline by sharing the very profound and transformative experiences that may occur while under the influence of these substances, many of which have been used as sacraments in religious and spiritual ceremonies for millennia to heal and connect with the divine. Through these incredibly powerful stories, this book series hopes to humanize these medicines and reintroduce their importance to mankind.

Disclosure

The sole purpose of *The Psychedelic Anthology* is to share people's real-life experiences with different psychedelic substances. In doing so, the creator of this book is not condoning, encouraging, or recommending their use and shall not be held liable or accountable for any loss, injury, or damage allegedly arising from the reading or discussing of this book's content. Furthermore, it is important to understand that the use of the substances mentioned in this book may lead to psychological or physical harm if used irresponsibly or improperly. As a reader, please be aware that the legality of the psychedelic substances discussed herein varies, and in different municipalities the possession, sale, or use of these substances may lead to fine or imprisonment.

Cover Art "Healer" by Heather McLean
www.hbomb.ca

Library of Congress Control Number: 2016955613
Copyright © 2016 by Aeternum, LLC. All rights reserved.

ISBN: 978-0-692-76376-6

To
Trust

A special thanks to **Shroomery.org** and all of the contributors for sharing their experiences.

APPENDIX

The
Psychedelic
Anthology

Volume I

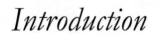
Introduction

THE MOST BEAUTIFUL DEATH

The following story consists of excerpts from a letter written by Laura Huxley, wife of psychedelic pioneer Aldous Huxley, about his experience with LSD on his deathbed and leading up to his final moments on November 22, 1963.

There is so much I want to tell you about the last week of Aldous' life and particularly the last day. What happened is important not only for us close and loving but it is almost a conclusion, better, a continuation of his own work, and therefore it has importance for people in general... It seemed obvious and transparent that subconsciously he knew that he was going to die. But not once consciously did he speak of it. This had nothing to do with the idea that some of his friends put forward, that he wanted to spare me. It wasn't this, because Aldous had never been able to play a part, to say a single lie; he was constitutionally unable to lie.

During the last two months I gave him almost daily an opportunity, an opening for speaking about death, but of course this opening was always one that could have been taken in two ways – either towards life or towards death, and he always took it towards life. We read the entire manual of Dr. Leary extracted from The Book of the Dead. He could have, even jokingly said don't forget to remind me his comment instead was only directed to the way Dr. Leary conducted his LSD sessions, and how he would bring people, who were not dead, back here to this life after the session. It is true he said sometimes phrases like, "If I get out of this," in connection to his new ideas for writing, and wondered when and if he would have the strength to work. His mind was very active and it seems that this Dilaudid had stirred some new layer which had not often been stirred in him.

"If I die." This was the first time that he had said that with reference to now. He wrote it. I knew and felt that for the first time he was looking at this. About a half an hour before I had called up Sidney Cohen, a psychiatrist who has been one of the leaders in the use of LSD. I had asked him if he had ever given LSD to a man in this condition. He said he had only done it twice actually, and in one case it had brought up a sort of reconciliation with death, and in the other case it did not make any difference. I asked him if he would advise me to give it to Aldous in his condition. I told him how I had offered it several times during the last two months, but he always said that he would wait until he was better. Then Dr. Cohen said, "I don't know. I don't think so. What do you think?" I said, "I don't know. Shall I offer it to him?" He said, "I would offer it to him in a very oblique way, just say 'what do you think about taking LSD [sometime again]?'" This vague response had been common to the few workers in this field to whom I had asked, "Do you give LSD in extremes?" *Island* is the only definite reference that I know of. I must have spoken to Sidney Cohen about nine-thirty. Aldous' condition had become so physically painful and obscure, and he was so agitated he couldn't say what he wanted, and I couldn't understand.

Then I don't know exactly what time it was, he asked for

his tablet and wrote, "Try LSD 100 intramuscular." Although as you see from this photo static copy it is not very clear, I know that this is what he meant. I asked him to confirm it. Suddenly something became very clear to me. I knew that we were together again after this torturous talking of the last two months. I knew then, I knew what was to be done. I went quickly into the cupboard in the other room where Dr. Bernstein was, and the TV which had just announced the shooting of Kennedy. I took the LSD and said, "I am going to give him a shot of LSD, he asked for it." The doctor had a moment of agitation because you know very well the uneasiness about this drug in the medical mind. Then he said, "All right, at this point what is the difference." Whatever he had said, no "authority," not even an army of authorities could have stopped me then. I went into Aldous' room with the vial of LSD and prepared a syringe. The doctor asked me if I wanted him to give him the shot – maybe because he saw that my hands were trembling. His asking me that made me conscious of my hands, and I said, "No I must do this." I quieted myself, and when I gave him the shot my hands were very firm. Then, somehow, a great relief came to us both. I believe it was 11:20 when I gave him his first shot of 100 microgrammes. I sat near his bed and I said, "Darling, maybe in a little while I will take it with you. Would you like me to take it also in a little while?" I said a little while because I had no idea of when I should or could take it, in fact I have not been able to take it to this writing because of the condition around me. And he indicated "yes." We must keep in mind that by now he was speaking very, very little. Then I said, "Would you like Matthew to take it with you also? And he said, "Yes." "What about Ellen?" He said, "Yes." Then I mentioned two or three people who had been working with LSD and he said, "No, no, basta, basta." Then I said, "What about Jinny?" And he said, "Yes," with emphasis. Then we were quiet. I just sat there without speaking for a while. Aldous was not so agitated physically. He seemed – somehow I felt he knew, we both knew what we were doing, and this has always been a great relief to Aldous. I have seen him at times during his illness very upset until he knew what he was going to do, then even if it was an operation or X-ray, he would make a total change. This enormous feeling of relief would come to him, and he wouldn't be worried at all about it, he would say let's do it, and we would go to it and he was like a liberated man. And now I had the same feeling – a decision had been made, he made the decision again very quickly. Suddenly he had accepted the fact of death; he had taken this moksha medicine (LSD) in which he believed. He was doing what he had written in *Island*, and I had the feeling that he was interested and relieved and quiet.

After half an hour, the expression on his face began to change a little, and I asked him if he felt the effect of LSD, and he indicated no. Yet, I think that a something had taken place already. This was one of Aldous' characteristics. He would always delay acknowledging the effect of any medicine, even when the effect was quite certainly there, unless the effect was very, very strong he would say no. Now, the expression of his face was beginning to look as it did every time that he had the moksha medicine, when this immense expression of complete bliss and love would come over him. This was not the case now, but there was a change in comparison to what his face had been two hours ago. I let another half hour pass, and then I decided to give him another 100 microgrammes. I told him I was going to do it, and he acquiesced. I gave him another shot, and then I began to talk to him. He was very quiet now; he was very quiet and his legs were getting colder; higher and higher I could see purple areas of cynosis. Then I began to talk to him, saying, "Light and free," Some of these thing I told him at night in these last few weeks before he would go to sleep, and now I said it more convincingly, more intensely – "go, go, let go, darling; forward and up. You are going forward and up; you are going towards the light. Willing and consciously you are going, willingly and consciously, and you are doing this beautifully; you are doing this so beautifully – you are going towards the light; you are going towards a greater love; you are going forward and up. It is so easy; it is so beautiful. You are doing it so beautifully, so easily. Light and free. Forward and up. You are going towards Maria's love with my love. You are going towards a greater love than you have ever known. You are going towards the best, the greatest love, and it is easy, it is so easy, and you are doing it so beautifully." I believe I started to talk to him – it must have been about one or two o'clock. It was very difficult for me to keep track of time. The nurse was in the room and Rosalind and Jinny and two doctors – Dr. Knight and Dr. Cutler. They were sort of far away from the bed.

I was very, very near his ears, and I hope I spoke clearly and understandingly. Once I asked him, "Do you hear me?" He squeezed my hand. He was hearing me. I was tempted to ask more questions, but in the morning he had begged me not to ask any more questions, and the entire feeling was that things were right. I didn't dare to inquire, to disturb, and that was the only question that I asked, "Do you hear me?" Maybe I should have asked more questions, but I didn't.

Later on I asked the same question, but the hand didn't move any more. Now from two o'clock until the time he died, which was five-twenty, there was complete peace except for once. That must have been about three-thirty or four, when I saw the beginning of struggle in his lower lip. His lower lip began to move as if it were going to be a struggle for air. Then I gave the direction even more forcefully. "It is easy, and you are doing this beautifully and willingly and consciously, in full awareness, in full awareness, darling, you are going towards the light." I repeated these or similar words for the last three or four hours. Once in a while my own emotion would overcome me, but if it did I immediately would leave the bed for two or three minutes, and would come back only when I could dismiss my emotion. The twitching of the lower lip lasted only a little bit, and it seemed to respond completely to what I was saying. "Easy, easy, and you are doing this willingly and consciously and beautifully – going forward and up, light andfree, forward and up towards the light, into the light, into complete love." The twitching stopped, the breathing became slower and slower, and there was absolutely not the slightest indication of contraction, of struggle. It was just that the breathing became slower – and slower – and slower, and at five-twenty the breathing stopped.

I had been warned in the morning that there might be some upsetting convulsions towards the end, or some sort of contraction of the lungs, and noises. People had been trying to prepare me for some horrible physical reaction that would probably occur. None of this happened, actually the ceasing of the breathing was not a drama at all, because it was done so slowly, so gently, like a piece of music just finishing in a sempre piu piano dolcemente. I had the feeling actually that the last hour of breathing was only the conditioned reflex of the body that had been used to doing this for 69 years, millions and millions of times. There was not the feeling that with the last breath, the spirit left. It had just been gently leaving for the last four hours. In the room the last four hours were two doctors, Jinny, the nurse, Rosalind Roger Gopal – you know she is the great friend of Krishnamurti, and the directress of the school in Ojai for which Aldous did so much. They didn't seem to hear what I was saying. I thought I was speaking loud enough, but they said they didn't hear it. Rosalind and Jinny once in a while came near the bed and held Aldous' hand. These five people all said that this was the most serene, the most beautiful death. Both doctors and nurse said they had never seen a person in similar physical condition going off so completely without pain and without struggle.We will never know if all this is only our wishful thinking, or if it is real, but certainly all outward signs and the inner feeling gave

13

indication that it was beautiful and peaceful and easy. And now, after I have been alone these few days, and less bombarded by other people's feelings, the meaning of this last day becomes clearer and clearer to me and more and more important. Aldous was, I think (and certainly I am) appalled at the fact that what he wrote in *Island* was not taken seriously. It was treated as a work of science fiction, when it was not fiction because each one of the ways of living he described in *Island* was not a product of his fantasy, but something that had been tried in one place or another and some of them in our own everyday life. If the way Aldous died were known, it might awaken people to the awareness that not only this, but many other facts described in *Island* are possible here and now. Aldous' asking for moksha medicine while dying is a confirmation of his work, and as such is of importance not only to us, but to the world. It is true we will have some people saying that he was a drug addict all his life and that he ended as one, but it is history that Huxleys stop ignorance before ignorance can stop Huxleys.

Even after our correspondence on the subject, I had many doubts about keeping Aldous in the dark regarding his condition. It seemed not just that, after all he had written and spoken about death, he should be left to go into it unaware. And he had such complete confidence in me – he might have taken it for granted that had death been near I certainly would have told him and helped him. So my relief at his sudden awakening at his quick adjusting is immense. Don't you feel this also?

Now, is his way of dying to remain our, and only our relief

and consolation, or should others also benefit from it? What do you feel?

Retrieved from www.lettersofnote.com/2010/03/most-beautiful-death.html

The
Experiences

SOMA, THE SPIRIT OF THE MUSHROOM

Psilocybin

"Mushroom spores are microscopic, beyond human and animal language, hard as diamonds and can travel in a vacuum from one planet to the next transforming rock into soil for biological life." – Roy Eskapa

As events and feelings have become infused with greater clarity over the past few weeks, I've come to understand my encounter with Soma as one of the most profound experiences of my life. I'm left with the sense that so much of my own journey has been leading up to this moment: that Soma has been waiting until I was ready to meet her. By the time I came, it was as if she had been expecting me.

I felt apprehension when I first arrived at Monica's house. I was in an unfamiliar place filled with new faces, and I began to doubt if I really knew what I was doing. Not eating all day added to my tension, and the stretch of time that passed between arriving at the house and taking the sacrament seemed protracted. I was quickly put at ease as each person introduced themselves and their intention. Everybody instantly became a relatable human with their own fears and vulnerabilities, their own past hurts and future hopes. Everyone in that room was just like me, and yet so utterly different and special and unlikely.

With all of our different stories, I soon recognized the people here as pilgrims on the path of self-knowledge. They had come in the pursuit of truth; they had come to heal and to transform, to know themselves and shatter the built up illusions of a society, culture, and civilization.

Soon after, we drank the tea infused with three different strands of Psilocybin mushrooms. The recommended dosage is no less than 5 grams. I can't say exactly, but it seemed like not even ten minutes had gone by before I began to feel something strange. My eyes became heavy and my body felt light. I remember a moment of enteral panic that screamed something like "Whoaaaa! No, no… NO! This is going to be way too intense! What am I doing? I don't want to go here! I want to turn back, which way do I turn back?" Another voice responded almost simultaneously. It spoke calmly as the voice of reason and it was the part of me that understood that I no longer had any control of where this journey was going, but I'd better just get on board and trust the direction because I wasn't going back. As this reality settled, my mind grew gentler and softer until all of my resistance disappeared completely. I surrendered, and with that my journey began to unfold.

As I moved deeper inside myself I felt an overwhelming sense of safety and trust for what was happening. I know that words, if not used well, can demystify what is experienced as sacred. Even attempting to form words and sentences over this experience seems an impossible task, but I feel it is still important to try.

I remember hearing a soft, gentle whisper. I first attributed this voice to Monica or one of the other guides looking after us that night, but each time I opened my eyes expecting to see one of them watching me, comforting me, no one was nearby. In that moment I began to recognize the divine voice of Soma. "You're just so tired, child. It's okay to rest now. Go to sleep," Soma whispered. My body began to unfurl and loosen itself. I became still and relaxed and I started to experience my mind as a single point of awareness. With this pure focus as my guide, I began to sink into the crevices of my own consciousness.

My journey began as a gentle unraveling of being, a stripping of all the insincerities and masks I had collected, a shattering of my assumptions, and a reaffirming of my neglected, exhausted dreams. I journeyed through great big galaxies and through great big wounds that felt as ancient as the Ice Age. I sat inside myself – my loneliness and my fear – and I acknowledged with compassion the frightened little girl inside of me. I began to see myself through gentle and loving eyes. All of my human perceptions and constructs diffused and I found myself floating through uncountable heavens. In this divine realm of compassion and kindness I saw kindred spirits all around me: the friends held closest, the poets and the music makers, angels, godheads, and cosmic playmates. I was dissolved, I was infinite, I was home. I felt myself soaring between great big masses of primordial rock adorned with faces that appeared as celestial beings and deities. In another moment I was swimming through a lake made of stars, realms that existed a trillion light years away yet lay at the core of my inner world. Nowhere in any of those deep corners did I find an infestation of fear. Fear – that sloppy, unwanted guest who won't leave the house of our everyday lives.

Every so often I'd force my eyes open just to be sure I was still on this planet. It was as if I was a submarine traveling into the deep, unexplored ocean of my unconscious mind, coming back to the surface of the water just to check I hadn't drowned. Everybody was still sitting around the room just like before. The painted ceiling was still above me, softly moving in beautiful pinks and greens. The hanging instruments and geometrics that filled the room appeared suspended as symbols of great power and truth. I looked over and saw Aikiko who had come from Japan, still beautifully poised and upright. I saw Ana in the corner, looking for a space to catch her tears. Opposite me I saw a mother whose eighteen-year-old daughter was on her own journey a few cushions away. The physical world was still intact, and I felt it an incredible reckoning to discover that all of the astral dimensions I was weaving through expanded across the plains of my own mind.

The journey passed through an entire spectrum of emotion. My core was set alight with a laughter that vibrated silently throughout my whole body, until the ecstasy and relief of it eventually brought me to tears. I remember wiggling my toes like a child wanting to dance, ecstatic in the music. I felt the divinity of my own nature, but most profoundly I felt it as the nature of every other being. I was washed with love for everyone in that room, everyone I had ever known, and everyone I would never actually meet. I imagined them in all their glory and beauty and it elated me. An immense feeling of gratitude flowed out of me. I became acutely aware of the brilliance of life, and I was experiencing it through the distillation of my thoughts into complex liquid patterns, by unfolding into moon lagoons and synthesizing into forested planets. I felt myself evaporating into the cool, dark, comforting atmosphere of the cosmos.

Soon the lessons would begin to take form and I knew I had to observe deeply and with trust in order to receive the messages that Soma was sending. I felt my experience as specific to my own story and yet it was entirely connected and intertwined with everybody else in the room. When Ana was weeping, I began to feel a rooted empathy for the pain she seemed to be carrying. I could see that part of me that was in her; I felt her experience as my own experience, her suffering as my suffering, and her tears as my own. I came face-to-face with that hurt and grieving child who also lived somewhere inside of me. I was presented with contrasting worlds and left with a choice of which one I would choose to inhabit.

I observed the world of fear, a world polluted by ignorance and assumptions, a world built from the fragile foundations of insecurity and worry. This was where wars were waged and promises were made out of the mouths of insincere lips. This world was layered with illusion and the hatred that caused suffering and confusion. This was a world we had been conditioned to live in our whole lives. It tore at us, at our hearts and our dreams and our land, until we thought less of those things than we did of each other.

As I scanned through the debris of this world, I began to see how little of it was actually real. We were so convinced of this superficial world, and our belief in it made us suffer. Life was so much bigger than any individual human story. It was bigger than all of the manufactured objects and dramas we played out over personal stages, across battlefields and borders, inside parliaments and prisons, and in front of the TV screens. I saw life as an ancient intelligence that moves, shifts, and evolves at a frequency of great beauty and divinity, its vibration penetrating through all of space. When we choose to live in the world of illusions we are trapped in the messy web of ignorance and Ego. We build constructs called religion, private ownership, development, national security, and race, and then go to war with each other and ourselves for the sake of those constructs. The illusion becomes more real than forests and rivers, more real than clean water and air, more real than blood and bones. We build outwardly in order to gain power in this fragile world. We try to gain security within an insecure structure, but a species can never be truly secure in an environment like that. You can never really win if you're the only one winning. We do it through our careers, through our possessions, by owning people and things. I began to mourn for the destruction of our Earth and for a humanity suffocating from illusion.

Just like a mother, Soma comforted me as I wept. She told me that it was alright, that it was okay to be here, and that all the wounds that left me frustrated, agitated, exhausted, and unconvinced could heal. This act of weeping felt sacred. It was my own confrontation of our collective suffering that I somehow always felt ingrained in and weighed heavy on my soul. I felt very strongly in that moment that if I could heal, our humanity would be able to heal too. "It's alright, go deeper into yourself,"

Soma whispered. So I went, feeling safe and suspended and supported. I wept for my family and the people I loved. I wept for my own ignorance. I mourned for the ravaging of the Earth and for the all weary, troubled hearts trapped at its surface.

In a strange and surprising way, Soma seemed to respond to my grieving with gratitude. I recognized Soma as the vibration that runs through all of life, as the bridge between our world and the hallowed land of dreams, as the Mother Earth, the mother we were forgetting. She was thankful that I cried for her. My awareness began to travel to those parts of my body that were stiff and numb or experienced drawn-out discomfort. Focusing on my left arm, the arm that carries my heart line, I had the sensation of an energy moving through me, unraveling my tension as though it was moving through the dormant passages of my body and clearing out the dead weight, making space for life and for the flow of the dancing waterfall.

I felt the beginning of geological time inside of my own body, as if the making of our galaxy had all been recorded there. I sensed the crashing of the Earth's tectonic plates and I slid between the melting of the Ice Ages into desert plains. Utterly ancient, I could feel the expansion of the Universe inside of me. That weeping was my letting go.

After a few hours I felt restless, so I got up and went outside. I fumbled towards the fire where some other people were sitting. I felt a discomfort rising in me, an insecurity, a kind of shyness. Perhaps it was because I was in the middle of a profoundly intimate experience with the Self, that I was still going through it and vulnerable in my deconstruction. Perhaps I was picking up on somebody else's experience completely different to my own, not knowing what anyone was dealing with or which thoughts they might be battling through in their own solitude and silence. I could never say for sure and whatever the reason was, I just let it be. I had no further reaction or comment. I had no defense or explanation to myself or to the others around me. I just allowed it to pass through me and did not allow it to possess me. A few seconds later, I was ready to move on freely.

I left the fire and went to look at the night sky. I saw the stars and planets with such intensity. I saw them shooting and burning, moving across the dark lacquer sky. I could see the pattern of how each star was connected. The connection appeared as a fractal flower in a dimension that had not been visible to me before. The stars seemed to rain on me and I knew that I was also a part of their beautiful web. The understanding was sublime. To experience these two moments in succession, fumbling through the fog of self-doubt to resolute clarity of my place in the Universe was an important lesson. I thought a lot about personal agency, about the frequency we choose to listen to, and it revealed how our thoughts are the precursors to our actions and the reality we create. Our thoughts become the way we see the world and ourselves. This was a constant practice of awareness and self-nurturing, and I was reminded that we have to choose it.

To journey into the realm of Soma is to undergo a journey of learning, disentangling, remembering, and healing. It is a place to marvel and explore, but it is never a place where you can escape. Each ecstatic insight or sensation needs to be carried back and lived in this world where we are intended to be at this moment, instead of getting lost forever in another time and place. At some point you have to say, "Okay, I better feed myself now," then get up to get a bowl of soup to ground yourself, even when you feel naked, exposed, and revealed. At some point you have to say, "I recognize the divine within me and I'm going to honor it by looking after my human needs and the human needs of others." Now, my normally quickened heart rate has slowed down, my breaths are deeper and calmer, and I sleep much better because I'm aware of the space that worry takes up. I try to only worry about things in the proper place and every moment of life feels more sacred than before.

We are so often bound by our narrow senses that we are always failing to see the connections of every thought and every action. We get glimpses of that truth sometimes through music, meditation, or drugs. But for the most part we choose to remain insensitive. We shouldn't forget the authentic nature of reality even when it is not always visible to our limited human senses. To remember its infinite intelligence and rapturous beauty is to exist in a state of playful grace.

Psychedelic explorer Terence McKenna was one of humanity's great crusaders of consciousness. After countless psychic explorations, he came to describe himself as the mouthpiece for the mushroom, relaying its messages and wisdom between our world and theirs. He once said: "Nature loves courage. You make the commitment and nature will respond to that commitment by removing impossible obstacles. Dream the impossible dream and the world will not grind you under, it will lift you up. This is the trick. This is what all these teachers and philosophers who really counted, who really touched the alchemical gold, this is what they understood. This is the shamanic dance in the waterfall. This is how magic is done. By hurling yourself into the abyss and discovering it's a feather bed."

WONDER FROM WITHIN

Psilocybin

As someone who has only ever previously altered their reality by use of alcohol, Cannabis, or prescribed toxins, psychedelics were that of an unknown realm to me. Having been a victim to fierce propaganda, I was falsely under the impression that psychedelics were only used by early twenty-something year old festival goers in search of a heightened experience or residual deadheads from the 70's. In my recent search for therapeutic alternatives regarding my own depression and anxiety, I came upon hard science from dedicated professionals that shed light on the beneficial aspects of some psychedelic experiences. As I came across more and more studies and personal experiences, I felt it was the missing piece to my healing.

My first experience with psychedelics was through about 2 grams of Psilocybin. Before I decided to dig deeper into my consciousness, I did a fair amount of research and asked trusted friends about their experience, but nothing could ever prepare me for what I was about to encounter.

The setting was just right: a small group of five in a texturally and visually appealing hotel room with incredible music. As we sat down together, we shared our intentions for the trip with each other. For myself, my intention was to truly allow myself to let go and let the fungi do its work. I reminded myself not to resist its hold as I began to feel the come up. I fought my Ego long enough to allow a wave of euphoria and love to wash over me. I felt warm and tingly, as if I could feel every blood cell rushing through my body. As I began to trust the fungi even more, I was able to tap into a reality I had never known existed. The visualizations started off mild as I watched the wallpaper pattern align with my heartbeat and begin to come alive. The lights pulsated and my body began to slip away from me. I watched in awe as faces and shapes began to take life. Ordinary objects were all of a sudden magical and I felt a sense of childhood wonder that I hadn't felt in years.

Needless to say, I found utopia at the bottom of an ice bucket. At the height of the trip each song seemed to catapult me into a totally different world from the last. One song in particular brought me spiraling head first into eternal pain, that of which I still have trouble fully understanding. The song resembled that of an earthy, indigenous drumming and chanting, almost ceremonial in nature. At that point, I had the urge to lie down and settle into the intense wave of emotions I was on the verge of experiencing. I chose a large red couch next to my fiancé and laid down, beginning to feel my body melt into the furniture. The fabric that was made of nylon and cotton transformed into the thickest, warmest, reddest blood I had ever seen. As I laid there in the strange blood, I felt immense sorrow and pain.

I closed my eyes and began to see vivid imagery of a lush rainforest surrounded by beautiful plants and animals. At the center of this forest, there was a giant, centuries-old tree and I found myself curled in a fetal position at its trunk. As my flesh melded with the wood of the tree, I could hear every drop of blood that had ever been spilled on this Earth. Names of people who have perished began to flash rapidly before my eyes. Some of which were familiar, but others I had never seen before. I allowed myself in that moment to truly feel pain, something I was scared of in my unaltered conscious state. I began to weep. I wept for anyone that had ever suffered and anyone currently still suffering.

As I wept in deep despair, I was presented with a divine feminine Spirit, an incredibly maternal love, as if to guide me through the darkest moments. While preparing for my experience, I compiled a list of questions I hoped to be answered. One of them regarded past lives. As I asked the Spirit who I was in a previous life, she seemed to scoff at my question, as if to say, "Here you are, presented in front of the Source and you ask me this?!" As I recoiled like a child being scorned, she relayed an incredible message to me: "You are everyone that has been and everyone that will be..."

At that moment, for the first time in twenty-nine years, I had the ability to understand what it was to be one, to be connected with one another as we truly are. As I was comforted by the notion of oneness, I began to apologize for myself and for all of humanity. The Spirit acknowledged my intentions and I was met with total and unconditional forgiveness. The Spirit reassured me that mankind still has time to make it right. I found, and still find, comfort in that thought as she left me alone in that tree trunk in the forest.

To many, my experience would be considered a bad trip. In spite of the intense pain and sorrow I was shown, deep down there was always a bright light full of hope. As I reflected on my experience during the come down, and weeks after, I viewed life and what I'm fighting for as an activist a little differently. I was able to have more compassion and empathy for others, knowing that others are doing their best finding their own path. I understood suffering is at the root of global unrest – the same suffering that could potentially be eliminated by use of natural medicine if there wasn't an outright war on consciousness.

It's safe to say I didn't realize the power of a mild dose of Psilocybin mushrooms. It has truly altered my reality forever and I am incredibly grateful for the lessons I have learned. Although I cannot say whether the therapeutic use of psychedelics is for everyone, I do believe it can benefit those who have exhausted their efforts to gain a better understanding of themselves. There isn't a self-help book, doctor, or pill that allowed me to gain the insight I have received from psychedelics, and for that I am truly grateful.

NATURE AND ITS GOLDEN HAND

LSD + MDMA + Ketamine

I was across the world in the country of Thailand and wound up on the rainforest island Koh Phangan for several nights. I made many friends there, mostly European, who spent their nights in a completely alternative reality than Western life – in fact, in an entirely separate community, built upon psychedelic experiences and open-minded love. I became entangled with this group of people, including an ex-love of mine who had transitionally moved to the island to escape the modern world of industrialization, destruction, and war indefinitely. This ex-love of mine happened to be someone that I had shared deep, profound psychedelic experiences with before. If I had to put him on a scale of meaning in my life, he would be considered one of my soul mates. We barely slept for five days when we saw each other again on the island. Wakefulness carried such light-bearing beauty that we did not want to miss a moment of the island together and did not feel the necessity of sleep.

This is an example of how powerful the mind is. The island itself had power to it and there was such a connection with nature, which showed me visions of its power before the substances were even involved. The deeper I went into nature, the more intimately I danced with the concepts of life and death, and "God reality." In my own poetic understanding, the messages I received from the Universe were, "You want to dance with me, here in nature. You will dance with me in beauty, but I will show you my power, because I am God. And the closer you are to God, the more I will bestow my power onto you as a light-bearer. But I will always choose who lives and who dies, and the closer you get to understanding, the closer you are to leaving this realm." Poetry is the only way to express these visions because it had been more of enlightenment than anything; a whole body and soul experience involving light, images, sensation of "knowingness," and words captured from the vines of nature.

After the introduction of psychedelics, this profoundness went to the next level. The psychedelics had been consumed multiple days in a row, with ebbs and flows of pinnacles in this river of life. To remain anonymous, I will not be using names in the story. Just know that when I had taken my first dose, I had been in a group of five people, three of which I shared prior intimate connections with, spiritually and emotionally. I became the light-bearer in our psychedelic experience. I guided the others into my spirit world, which was filled with insight of the oneness and interconnectedness to God, nature, and soul. We felt the triumphing power of the Universe engulf us, which is far vaster. The five of us were handed an overwhelming sensation of "knowingness." We were exactly where God wanted us, at the center of the Universe, engulfed by nature.

We found ourselves on a bed in our bungalow, which had the effect of feeling outdoors even when we were inside. We could hear the noises of the animals rustling around outdoors, and birds chirping. We could hear the raindrops falling from leaf to leaf, trees swaying in the wind, and thunderstorms passing through with gushes of electricity. Everything felt infinitely peaceful, as if the warmth in my soul radiated from the osteon of my bone to the eyelids catching the fresh air. We felt truly happy to be with each other. We all sat there, smiling at each other, understanding how nature enlightens and breathes life into humans when they dance more intimately with its spirit.

Our conversation on a bed, in a home overlooking the rainforest, became a table for discussion, with few words, but shared understanding. Our conversations became direct conversations with the Universe, guiding the fate of the current realm we reside in. In other words, we discussed the world through the eyes of God.

The following day we tripped again, and I carried the other four group members into an alternative dimension where the world in which we reside became completely irrelevant. I understood it had been me as the carrier because the more my mind, energy, and soul escalated, the more the five of us traveled into this psychedelic world. My friend turned to me acknowledging this, confirming "this ride is mine," and this friend came forward admitting how my mind took him on a journey in sobriety a few months later. I believe that my deeper connection to the spirit or natural world allowed me to carry the others through their experience and escalate its intensity. At one particular plateau, I traveled into a world in which there was no pain and suffering, only abstract concepts and ideas. The visions I received about this world were fractals of light, and this world multiplied indefinitely as if I were staring into an endless mirror – a tunnel of possibilities. Essentially, the concept that this world is not the last in our journey together had been demonstrated, and the infinite God had become overwhelmingly apparent. I knew I had been on the edge of another dimension – where God had been demonstrating to me how large and vast he, I, and we sentient beings are, which my mind stretched so far, it came full circle into another realization how we are all one together.

Again, I derived from the powers I had been shown that our current realm is extremely sensitive to our actions and projections and relies on human ingenuity to end human and natural world suffering. We are very much one with God when we allow ourselves to be, and although that is a fine line walking amongst the things we do not currently understand, it is a much more inviting experience than remaining in our ignorant, selfish, and "safe" yet poisonous worlds separate from true reality. In summary, I would rather walk that fine line of insanity than waste another day in fake reality. All in all, when life and death is walked with by God, it is welcoming with open arms.

Another peak had occurred during a night-time celebration with hundreds of ex-pats from all over the world, many of which were also consuming psychedelics. There had been a beautiful jagged rock overcasting the waves, which created tunnels and pockets for the ocean to release its rage. This landing had become an anchor site for the experience, where people gravitated toward its beauty in a circular fashion throughout the night. I personally found myself glued to this rock, because the stars and energy were intensifying, and the sky turned into an oil painting only the Universe and us sentient beings of love could have created. I found myself in tears of overwhelming beauty.

Our enlightenment and connection to God painted the sky in the most beautiful, overwhelming landscape of euphoria I could imagine. With a whole field of people dancing underneath the stars in this dream world of the wild and free, I felt it had been our rising of spirit into a world so much more divine than the 9-to-5 that created this atmosphere, and I felt the euphoria of heaven on Earth, with our willingness to accept dreams as reality. My mind became so large it raised the conscious awareness of everyone else around me. I knew I had found a special place in the heart of my soul. I found warmth and enlightenment, in people smiling as they should be – completely free.

During the sun rising, I noticed the atmosphere filled with people embodied into their truest form of self: the free spirit. All I could see was beautiful people and happiness running wild in nature. I could see no faults in the eyes of nature and living in accordance with nature's will. We spent an hour or so enjoying the sunlight rising into the skies, painting a dramatic transition from stars to sun.

We returned to the bungalow after sun rising, which upon arrival we decided to re-introduce Ketamine. The effects of MDMA wore off at this point, and we were still on LSD. Time and space split, and then split again, and again, and again... alone in the solitude of my mind, experiencing the infinite, in a place with no time, no boundaries, visually resembling a mirror facing another mirror. Suddenly, the abstract Universe became apparent.

Knowledge is larger than I, you, or the current level of consciousness, and I view this knowledge as "God Knowledge" slowly being extracted from our connection to nature and its will. The further away we separate from it, the further away we are from ending suffering. In one night, God demonstrated to me a power greater than us and the next demonstrated how vast the Universe is which I am a part of, infinitely, and which I dream to be bound to Nature, God, and its Golden Hand.

FEAR

Ayahuasca

It begins at the pit of the stomach, and then it spreads to the rest of the body. There is a sense of restlessness, agitation, and an inability to concentrate. At times, it would actually paralyze me. I felt a strong desire to flee it somehow, a desire to stop the discomfort. Yet it won't leave me. In the past I would have found ways to distract myself; call someone, listen to music, eat something, watch TV, anything to keep me from feeling this disturbing energy living inside of me. Sometimes, I would actually stop and listen to it. I would go inside and attempt to get to the source of these experiences. Other times, just redirecting my attention to them would alleviate their intensity. Although, most of the time they would get more severe and cause me to flee again. However, I discovered that avoiding or distracting myself from them clearly did not diminish them or make them disappear. On the contrary, the faster I ran, the stronger they got. The pain became so unbearable that I could no longer avoid the simple truth: there is no place to run. It finally dawned on me – these feelings are mine. They live in me. They are part of me. Running away from them only meant running away from myself.

I made the decision not to run anymore. It was time to take responsibility for all of my experiences, external and internal. It was time for me to become acquainted with these feelings and understand why they were there. They were mine, and I needed to learn about them. I needed to learn about myself. Let me be perfectly clear, this was not an easy decision. I arrived at it only when I became aware that the pain of avoiding these feelings was worse than the feelings themselves. Owning them was a huge breakthrough for me. Understanding and accepting that the source of these feelings was inside of me and that I needed to go within rather than outside of me in order to relieve them was my first step toward appreciating their value.

The process was and remains uneven. It is a constant challenge for me to go into this discomfort zone. When the feelings arise, my first inclination is still to flee, and sometimes I do, though not for long. It takes great effort, but I am now able to remind myself to stop and listen. I force myself to sit still and quiet. Using my consciousness, I enter my body and sweep over it. I notice where I am tight, where I am jittery, where I am confused, and how every part of my being wants to distract me. Over time, as I began to listen more intently, I started hearing the fear. My mind would be chattering about some possible failure, some horrible mistake, or some potential wrongdoing. The content could be about something that happened in the past or something related to a future decision or event. Feelings of insecurities, judgments about what I am doing versus what I should be doing, or worries about how things may turn out bombard my mind. Initially, this led to my feeling more overwhelmed and confused, intensifying the desire to escape them. But my commitment to be with everything inside me inspires me to stay put and continue the process.

As I reflect on what I have written thus far, what I recognize is the manner in which the past and the present tenses seem to merge together. In the world of emotions there is no past or present, there is only the now. And often the now of the emotions is the single existing reality. If I am in joy, I can hardly relate to a feeling of sorrow and when I am in pain I cannot relate to being happy. The emotional world has the capacity to grab all of my attention and focus it only on that which I am feeling. Consequently, when I experience pain or sorrow, it is as if I am falling into this never-ending space from which I cannot break away. Because my emotions are so powerful and all encompassing, when bringing attention to them, I actually feel like I am going to get stuck there – hence my desire to flee.

I am fleeing because when I am inside them I don't see a way out. The pain gets more painful, the fear becomes greater and the agitation and irritability increases. Any attempts to conjure up other feelings fail miserably. The experience is one of absolute loss, aloneness, and darkness. Nothing is possible in this space; there is no escape. I feel helpless, vulnerable, and confused. My mind wants to fix these feelings. It wants to understand them and make them better. It begins to try to figure them out. It questions what is wrong with me and why I am feeling this way. It begins to torment me with criticism and judgment. It does not want these feelings there and it demands that I get rid of them somehow. NOW!! It goes around in circles, aggravating them further as it attempts to make sense of them and explain them away. As long as the mind does its thing, the emotions are doing theirs. As the mind attempts to distract, explain and suppress them, the emotions insist on remaining exactly where they are, and if anything they will fortify themselves and exaggerate themselves so that they will not be carelessly dismissed. They will be heard one way or another and there is nothing the mind can do about it. They want my undivided attention and they refuse to let the mind hijack my consciousness. They are here to communicate with me and they know they have something important to share with me.

The power of the emotions and their nature of being the only thing that exists in the moment overwhelm the mind. It is inconceivable to the mind that the emotions need to be surrendered to. Not seeing a way out, the mind wants to protect itself and my psyche from the never-ending pain it imagines. In the midst of the emotional experience, it has no clue that these emotions are temporary. It also has no clue that the emotions are more than just uncomfortable feelings, that they actually may hold information that is essential for my well-being. Therefore, it fights to protect itself and me from its perception of perpetual suffering. One may ask, "Why am I separating my mind from myself?" The fact is that I am not my mind, just as I am not my emotions. The "me" part of me – the conscious part of me – is not my mind, not my body, and not my emotions. Understanding that, reality helps me extricate myself from my mind's fears and distortions, as it reminds me that these feelings are just temporary and actually useful for me to explore. I am getting ahead of myself. More on this further ahead.

The struggle is arduous and downright excruciating. Appreciating the conflict is the first place to start. Understanding the dynamics helps me to remain present to the emotions and not succumb to the mind's chatter. I begin by listening to my emotions, listening with my consciousness, not my mind. I remain in my body, in spite of my mind's desire to distract me. I feel the pain, I feel the fear, I feel the helplessness, I feel the darkness, I feel the loneliness, I feel the heartbreak, I feel the sorrow, I feel the pain. It is getting deeper and deeper, it seems to be endless, the more I feel, the more I feel, the more I feel, the deeper I go, the deeper I go, the more lost I feel. The pain becomes unbearable. I feel the heat, I feel the terror, the darkness surrounds me, engulfs me, I am all alone, I am all alone. God help me. This is so scary. This is terrifying… I am all alone.

I AM ALL ALONE. This is where I invariably arrive. This is the darkness I am so petrified of experiencing. Here it is – the truth of this moment. It is masked in so many ways. It dresses itself in the many other garbs of emotions. All the fears, the insecurities, the pain, the sorrow, the anxieties, the conflicts, the stories, the shame, the worries, the grief, are all there to mask the bottom line, fear – I AM ALONE, I AM SEPARATE. I stand at the edge of this emotion, afraid to move one step forward. A sense of dread and paralysis comes over me. Where do I go from here? What am I to do now? How could this be? I want to go back, but go back to where? I just came from there and here I am. It is all the same. There is no turning back. I am all alone

The terror is unbearable. There is nothing in front of me. There is nothing behind me. There is nothing but darkness around me. I come face to face with the void. This is the abyss I'd been avoiding for so long. Where am I? Who am I? An unspeakable feeling of vulnerability comes over me. An overwhelming sense of helplessness, powerlessness, and confusion envelops me. It feels as if the ground has fallen from underneath my feet. I have lost my footing; my world has collapsed around me. Suddenly, I find myself gripping onto a rock by my fingers. I am dangling in this darkness, terrified, as I realize there is nothing I can do. My arms are getting tired. I hold on for dear life as the foreboding feeling of death comes over me. I am going to have to let go. My God, I am going to die. I am going to die. The pain is agonizing. The fear is paralyzing. No longer able to hold on, I SURRENDER. I let go into the darkness. I let go to my death. My body plummets deep into the vortex with an unimaginable force of gravity. As my body is falling, calmness comes over me. I begin to experience a different sense of awareness. My identification with my body fades away, my mind disappears, and my emotions vanish. All that is left is my consciousness, and it is now rising. No body, no mind, no emotions – no Ronit – just pure awareness.

This state of awareness seems fleeting as it floats in the darkness and abruptly merges with some powerful light source. Then there is nothing. Awareness arises again. Energy is everywhere. A consciousness of the Cosmos gives way to wholeness – to oneness. Everything is ever-present. There are vibrational frequencies everywhere. Forms arise as vibrations – trees, rocks, animals, humans, and objects, all vibrating their own frequencies – yet, all are sourced by the same energy force. It all fits together. Everything fits together – it is an interdependent whole.

With this full awareness, my consciousness re-enters my body. An overwhelming feeling of connectedness and love comes over me. A complete understanding of my relationship to the whole penetrated my every being. We are one! We are not separate. We are part of this great, intelligent energy force – we are part of spirit. There is no such thing as death. Our experience of death is merely an illusion of the mind – the mind that in its limited, temporal state perceives us as separate. Our consciousness is ever-present with our source.

The realization of our deep, existential experiences of aloneness and fear of death comes crushing down around me. I observe that all the suffering I experienced prior to my surrender was due to my fear of being alone; my fear of death. Had I known then what I know now, I would have let go immediately. I would have surrendered to the darkness of the abyss with absolute abandon. At once, I am filled with an extraordinary sense of sadness and compassion as I relieve the sensations of pain and terror that so overwhelmed me just before my surrender. I was present to both these excruciating emotions and the absolute awareness of their illusion. The sadness that came over me arose from my knowledge that until we surrender and experience the illusion of death, we inevitably will suffer the accompanying pain and terror. The compassion came from my connection with all of humanity and knowing first hand that this is a subjective, personal experience that everyone must go through and there is nothing I can say or do to alleviate their suffering.

I began to cry like I have never cried before. The depths of my feelings, as sad as they were, filled my heart with unimaginable warmth and unity. Clearly, I was tapping into the universal well of Love. Its power, its intensity, its goodness, and tenderness kept washing over me like waves in the ocean. I became submerged with its core, its essence, its truth. For the first time I realized what it means to be in love, that is, inside love. Love was not inside of me – I was inside love. I had arrived home. It is not as if I had to do anything or go anywhere. Love is always there. I am always in it whether I am conscious of it or not. All that happened for me is that I woke up to it. The veil of illusion was lifted to reveal where I have always been – where I am always.

I could feel my soul dancing, soaring, and laughing joyously. I am home; I have always been home. We are all home. An unspeakable yearning to share with others came over me. Where do I begin? What do I say? How can I communicate this experience, this knowledge? As Socrates said, "I cannot pour sight into eyes, they must see for themselves."

THE MIRACLE OF MIND LOSS

DMT

It didn't work very well when I heated it up in the bottle. A good amount of the vapor escaped out of the sides because I was kind of sloppy with the foil and the tape. There was still a small amount of vapor built up in the bottle, but I didn't feel like it was enough for me to get a good enough hit. So, my friend who initially wasn't going to do any DMT that night decided he'd try that small amount rather than waste what was already there. The way he inhaled it was slow and smooth, like he was drinking it out of the bottle. After he finished it, he lied back on the bed, closed his eyes, and stood very still. We asked him if he was feeling anything and he replied with, "I don't really understand it." A chill ran up my spine as he said that, knowing that while he certainly didn't break through, he was still feeling something that went beyond what our minds can understand. As he was lying down, I prepared my dose. When he came back, he said that he didn't have any kind of out-of-body experience, but he definitely did feel a presence. One that almost had a way of communicating that he wasn't ready at that moment.

I heated the substance up, watching as the bottle filled up with thick vapor, a good deal more than the first time. I figured it was filled enough, so after lying down on the bed I uncapped it and quickly inhaled. The harshness of the smoke hit me more than anything. I laid back and closed my eyes expecting to be thrown into hyperspace, but not much happened except my heart rate went up incredibly fast and I felt a very warm enveloping presence. It almost felt like it was telling me I was not ready yet. Behind my eyelids I saw shadows warp and contort but there was nothing colorful or anything that was really reminiscent of DMT. I could still hear the sounds of the room, the whispers of my friends, so I knew I didn't go anywhere. I opened my eyes and the room did have a different kind of glow to it. The lights were ever so gently warping or breathing but that was really it. Disappointed, I waited a full hour.

I gave in and began packing my friend's bubbler with herb, followed by a layer of DMT, followed by another top layer of herb. I meditated once again, gently breathing in through the nose and out through the mouth, reminding myself to surrender to the trip and to try to learn something. I got comfortable, laid back, took in one last deep breath, pressed the bubbler to my lips and began to gently light the top layer of bud. The flame just barely kissed the flower. I released the carb, and without removing my lips from the pipe, I let it milk up two or three times. I could taste the DMT and knew I was getting a really good hit. It really isn't that terrible when it's mostly being covered up with weed smoke. I held in the smoke when I was done and handed the pipe to my friend, who was next to me on the bed. Before I even exhaled I could already feel it working on my body. It sort of felt like I was being crushed at first and then the last thing I saw was my release of smoke into the room.

I could see reality being pushed back as I closed my eyes and

I heard my friends saying, "Take one more hit," but as soon as I closed my eyes it was too late. There was an electronic sound that resembled a computer "blip" and I was there instantly. I heard, or rather felt, an eerily sharp tone. As soon as I entered the space their voices got farther away and I was submerged. It felt like I had just leaped out of something and was dropping into a space that completely defied all the natural laws of physics I was accustomed to. The space was dark with a strong electric influence. The great McKenna could not have put it better: "The initial feeling is as though one has just been struck by noetic lightning."

It greatly resembled a holographic grid, wide open, no floor and no ceiling – just space. It felt like I was flying but falling at the same time, and I immediately started to see things of overwhelming beauty. The visuals started out very simple but they quickly changed, becoming infinitely more complex. At first I just saw straight colorful lines that rapidly turned into patterns, threads, and shapes that were intertwining, rotating, and morphing in an elegant dance of beautiful chaos. It is hard to remember specifics but I distinctly remember rotating cubes that were made of glowing pink and green light.

I began to hear electric symphonies echoing through this infinite hall of raw possibility. Music that made no sense, but was so beautiful and could never be replicated in our normal reality. The patterns danced perfectly to the sound of the music. Structures began forming out of the patterns. They were being sung into existence. Most of the structures looked like a cross between a pyramid and a castle along with many other cultural

49

hybrid structures.

My life did unfold before my eyes, but it was so quick that it was impossible to make sense of it or see any specific memories. I believe I saw the chrysanthemum that McKenna often spoke of. I saw some sort of an extremely rapidly rotating mandala or portal into infinity. Time was moving way too fast for me to keep up or understand what was happening. The space I was in was extremely abstract and very hard to comprehend. It was almost as if I was floating the entire time. I wish I could explain it but like most DMT concepts it's very hard to convey an articulate explanation of the experience. It felt as though I had entered into an extremely futuristic medical environment. Everything was made of this glowing blue-white crystal that mirrored how we use glass in modern architecture.

Next I was lying down and being operated on by these beings. They really had no faces or bodies or definition whatsoever but somehow they were still there. They were nothing more than a presence. I couldn't see them, but they were there, clear as anything else in life. Time was still moving at an incredibly fast rate, so I experience all of these medical procedures at a rate that just simply wasn't possible to pay attention to, as much as I wanted to. All I know is they were definitely injecting me, taking samples of whatever they needed, performing strange experiments with strange instruments, and finally cleaning what I believe was my soul.

I was receiving some kind of communication but I couldn't make sense out of most of it. I think that there were many of them but I was only able to communicate with one. It was a beautiful warm feminine presence. It wasn't like she was speaking to me using only her voice. There were other mediums being used, but I couldn't tell exactly what they were. When the beings communicated with me they were singing in an abstract language, releasing auditory vibrations like us, but they were also using visualizations and sensations that just can't be described. It went beyond words and beyond intellect. This strange transportation of information was so soft, kind, and gentle. She was telling me things like "It's all going to be alright," "You're doing very well with this," and "It will all be over soon."

The next thing I knew I was being thrusted in a direction I could only assume was up, and at this moment something very strange happened. I suddenly seemed to become synchronized with everything. Time stood still for a moment and I could perceive everything that exists, has existed, or will exist. It was so familiar and so overwhelming, and I knew I had experienced this an infinite number of times. I had been here before in this strange sensorium on mushrooms, but more importantly I had been here before between lives.

This is where you go when you die. It is where we all came from and it is where we will all return. I call it Source because I don't know what else to call it. It is the peak of existence, the pinnacle of creation, and the climax of evolution. It is the moment when my mind connects with the mind of the Sublime, enters the realm of the Interior, and experiences an alien miracle I call the Organic Divine. It is an intimate connection between me and the natural Universe.

In this mystical experience, all wisdom, magic, and possibility stewed together in a primordial ooze of oneness. It was both ancient and futuristic because it was where the beginning made love to the end and every moment in time blended together in this organized fluidity that erupted in an explosion of cosmic sexual energy. This overflow of sensation felt like an orgasm, but one that went above and beyond the physical, for it was an orgasm of spirit, not body. I would also describe this sensation as feeling like you are drowning, being born, dissolving into all which is, or even go as far as to say having sex with God.

These words don't even come remotely close to doing the experience justice. It is the most ineffable and astonishing moment that one simply cannot comprehend or conceive with a human mind. It doesn't make sense at all, but it's so god damn beautiful. It loves the fuck out of you and you love the fuck out of it. It is your True Self seeing itself in all things. This indescribable thing, this ultimate feeling became so overwhelming and then I blinked and was back in this room with three people that I think I know.

The room had no definition, very similar to a really old 8-bit video game. Everything was made of lines of red, turquoise, and white light, fractals, and eyes. I heard a sharp ringing going through my head and the static crackle of a radio tuner. I was being tuned back into reality. There was a big guy with long hair sitting in a computer chair and he was completely blacked out. His figure was just totally jet black, empty. I was extremely confused, disoriented, and incoherent. It felt like I had just been born into another world. Reality. I didn't remember that I was on a drug, who I was, or where I was. I very suddenly started to get paranoid, fearing that my "friends" were up to something. I thought perhaps they were planning on calling some kind of authority that would take me away to a psychiatric institution. I feared that I had gone completely insane. Crazy patterns that I couldn't describe if I tried started to form on the walls of the room, which was suddenly becoming more defined. Reality was reforming itself like a fucking puzzle before my very eyes. My Ego and identity were coming back to me. I was a human being from planet Earth who had just smoked DMT. I was proud of myself for knowing that.

Music began playing – a beautiful song that reminded me of my favorite LSD trip that took place on top of Cadillac Mountain, eventually ending up at Sand Beach when it was deserted at midnight. The music was distorted in some ways yet it sounded more clear and crisp than ever before. "I hear the drums echoing tonight, but she hears only whispers of some quiet conversation. She's coming in, 12:30 flight. Her moonlit wings reflect the stars that guide me towards salvation. I stopped an old man along the way, hoping to find some old forgotten words or ancient melodies. He turned to me as if to say, 'Hurry boy, it's waiting there for you.'"

It was all starting to come back to me. My friend was no longer blacked out. He gave me a bottle of water and as soon as I drank it I felt almost completely submerged back into reality. It felt like I had just floated back down to Earth; like I was reborn. I felt all of my fears and paranoia wash away, I literally felt wet. And then I finally understood that it was all going to be okay, that I was back in reality and had just been a part of something so indescribably beautiful and in a way that will always be.

I felt a deep love for my friends and for everything in the Universe; euphoria more powerful than anything I've experienced on any other drug. Everything looked so intricately fractal both with eyes open and closed. I still had incredible glowing visuals that I simply couldn't compare to the visuals I've had on either LSD or mushrooms. I guess they were almost like a blend of both but they were certainly unique all on their own. The visuals seemed to dance for me in the happiest way possible. The rug on the floor, which wasn't that interesting ordinarily, was arranged in a pattern that reminded me of the Grateful Dead bears. They were waving goodbye as if they were saying, "Bye! See you next time!"

NIRVANA AND HELL

5-MeO-DMT

Am I as scared to write this as I think I am? When I first wrote about DMT a few years ago, it took months for me to come to terms with the awe and find the words. I am only four days out from the most powerful event of my life, still scratching the bug bites from my days spent lying in the sand of Punta Chueca. Yes, I am afraid.

We had done an Ayahuasca ceremony the night before and were going on little sleep when we pulled into the secluded cove the day after the Full Moon. The doctor and Shaman whom I had met the night before were both there, holding rattles and a feather stick. My biggest concern was the scorching heat with only one application of sunscreen. A fellow psychonaut tried to divert my attention from the Ayahuasquero who had just smoked the 5-MeO and whose eyes were rolled back into his head with bubbles coming out of his mouth. She held me close to her and asked me to look only into her eyes. She said, "You go in there and be all that you ARE. You are magnificent. You are beautiful."

They held towels up around me to protect the flame from the wind. The doctor had me take several deep breaths and held the glass bulb pipe to my lips. "Slowly…" he cautioned. I sucked in the smoke and finished it only with his persistence. I told myself to hold it in as instructed, but I wanted to exhale.

I stood in the beautiful sun and my body almost immediately dissolved into white light. Like confetti, I fell apart. I lost myself completely and ceased to exist. I do not remember anything here, but was moving my arms quite a bit. I wonder if this is what they refer to as the "white out." The next thing I remember is not being human. I don't remember what was happening, but I know I was increasingly losing control. I was beginning to kick my legs and run in place, though I had collapsed on the ground. My throat sounds start low and gradually became higher-pitched and more afraid. Things began to turn inside out in ways that don't make sense at all. Every atom in my body was attacking me, and every dimension that ever made sense was imploding and taking me with it. I had no thought of Self or my name or my body or 5-MeO-DMT. I was gone completely, lost in ever-evolving agony. And I was more and more out of control. I didn't even have these thoughts. My essence was being twisted into all that is Hell and it only came on faster and more intensely. If I even attempted to find myself, I was punished with more horror and pain. I didn't even know the word "release" or the term "let go." I am in the grip of Hell itself – pain and horror that cannot be described here.

It is at this point the doctor turned me over on my back and my human body stopped breathing. My friend tells me my face had gone purple and that he saw the doctor become concerned. They poured water into my throat to get me to breathe for survival. In my Hell, the water they poured became another part of the madness and propelled me into farther, more isolated levels of Hell. I am drowning, I am dying. I am dying everyone's death, I am all the pain that ever has existed, and that's a silly understatement. I knew I was in very serious trouble and began to truly panic.

I suddenly saw myself clearly. I have finally done 5-MeO, the ultimate thing I've been so foolishly chasing, and I'm trapped. I am worse than insane. I am trapped in a Hell that is compounding upon itself infinitely with each unfolding moment. It cannot get worse... and then it does. Again and again. Shockingly. Disturbingly. Infinitely. Over and over and over until my sheer terror makes me crack wide open and accept it.

This is my new reality. The certainty is terrifying. I am the poster child for "the one who got lost forever," "the one who never came back," "the cautionary tale for all psychedelic users for the rest of time." They bring in Buddhist monks, healers, priests, and exorcists. No one could get me out. I assume peripherally that from the outside my head is shaking back and forth. I'm clawing my face, and screaming with all that I am. This is how I will look for the rest of time to the outside world. But inside my soul it will always only be this compounding, infinite horror. I'm left alone to act as the example. It's what my whole life has been leading to. I, ME, Jennifer... this has been my destiny all along. This is my purpose. I am the Chosen One to embody Hell for others to learn from. To the spiritual people of the world, the Burners and psychonauts, monks and yogis, I am a Legend, and they pay solemn homage. They speak about me at gatherings and try to make sense of me. They come see me, locked up in a museum with glass walls, living out my private Hell for them to observe. They cry and shake their heads. I make them shudder and have disturbing nightmares. Most are too afraid to come see me at all. I become a tragic relic.

As I fully accept this, my panic becomes so immense that I lose my mind. Complete psychosis. Absolute and desolate madness. I implode into the Hell that has become my only companion. If there were a boulder, and I was able to use my body, I would have smashed my head on it until death released me. With horror, I remind myself that this reality will not end with my death. I am trapped. Forever. The only True Lost Soul in the Universe. I am what everyone fears. Does that make me Satan? No. It makes me the opposite of Light. I am Darkness. The Yin. I am Suffering itself. The Chosen One trapped here to allow the other side to exist. It was ME all along. How's that for destiny? A single loud clap cuts through the compounding malevolence, and instantly, everything goes white...

Silent.

Still.

Am I dead?

I am nowhere.

It is so white.

The doctor begins singing one of his ancient songs. To be

honest, I am not sure what finally transitioned me to the Light, but I know his song is now the Arcana imprinted on my soul forever. I find myself humming it every moment my mind is quiet. I felt it through every minute of sleep last night. It guided me out of the darkness. At first I thought the doctor saved me, but now I am starting to believe I saved myself. I had to conquer Hell to reach Nirvana. The price was high. But you get what you pay for.

Surrender...?

Nirvana blooms into all existence. It is a soft, pastel, fractal of Being. Of oneness, of light, more than love. It is free of suffering and beyond the cycle of death and rebirth. I reach true Nirvana. True enlightenment. The beauty and reality and pureness of it is compounding equally as infinitely as Hell had before. It is equally intense. Building, yes, but also becoming more and more real. More true. I slowly realize that this Nirvana is not just within ME or something I've reached. All of existence now finds itself here for all eternity. The thought of wars crosses my mind, and I realize they are no more. All suffering has ceased. We are allowed to simply exist here now. Forever.

In the greatest moment I have ever known, it dawns on me that it has all come from ME. There has been a tiny hidden atom located behind my ribcage that has held the power all along. THIS is my destiny! I am the Chosen One to release all beings back into Nirvana. We have found our way home! And the same spiritual community of Burners and seekers now pay homage to the humble one who somehow held the key to unlock all of True Being. And they shake their heads in delight and amazement because no one could have guessed it would come from such a small person. We had all done our parts by awakening others, or feeling gratitude, or doing yoga, or fasting, or praying, or loving one another, or being patient with ourselves.

What we have all been seeking, I now fully realize I have found for us all. There are no "thank you's" – just infinite joy that it has come back around at last. Our hard work is over!! We all did it together! We did it! I am God in the existence of Nirvana, as are we all, and this knowledge validates all I have ever been and ever will be.

I have been dealing with some intense flashbacks of the difficult part, and I have been afraid to be alone. I'm having trouble relating to people and teachings that used to comfort me. The Arcana has really seemed to be my crutch, but I intend to release it soon. I can feel myself getting stronger. I believe now that I experienced a literal rebirth. My wonderful friend said to me, "Hell is no longer just a word to you. But then again, neither is Nirvana."

After writing all of this and reflecting in the past few days, I believe my takeaway is this: I am not lost. I am not trapped or doomed. I do not have to be afraid. I am not alone. I am all that exists. I am responsible for Nirvana, and I will always find my way back to the Light.

THE SHAMANIC JOURNEY WITHIN

Psilocybin

After taking down 7 grams of Plant Teachers, a strain of Psilocybin mushrooms, I sat amongst my brothers calling upon the IAM presence, The Golden Flame, The Emerald Flame, and The Violet Flame. I lied down with great joy and comfort as I began to enter meditation, for I feel my guides are near. As thoughts slowly passed by and faded, I was met by that oh-so-familiar world of living geometry and liquid flame. I perceived that which emanates throughout all of creation, that which animates all that is – the primal essence of sound and light at play.

As I observed this great beauty, an immensely soothing voice asked me a question, like a graceful host asking his honorable guest if he may nourish and grant him whatever he desires. "What do you wish to learn?" Within an instant it was made clear to me that this parenchymal plane of geometry was a library, a tissue that held information. This place is not separate from myself or anyone for that matter, for it is all that is. Overly ecstatic and overwhelmed thoughts arose again, "Whatever my heart desires? I can learn anything?" I told the heavenly host, "I greatly wish to further learn of my star history. Where has my soul been? What missions and journeys have I embarked on? What areas of the Universe have I traversed and transmigrated to and from and why?"

Suddenly, I was being pulled! The geometry that I perceived reacted as if it were excited I had asked this!! I became swallowed by a tunnel of portals, zooming at what felt like incredible face-shredding speeds into this multi-dimensional fractal universe of portals that led to universes of more portals. Somehow through this intense trip a thought slipped in. "Could this be what I learned as the Akashic libraries?" Simply because that one thought arose, a flood of thoughts came in and broke the pure observation. More and more questions came in and instead of me receiving the answers to the questions I had originally asked for; I was being pulled from portal to portal. It was as if my own overexcitement disrupted this intense experience.

The heavenly host asked once more, "Where do you wish to go and what do you wish to learn?" I answered instead this time with deep silence and immense reverence. No longer was I separate from these great mysteries. No longer did I desire to reach for anything. I surrendered, and all that was left was my Being. Upon this great surrender, I felt that which was "Michael" unravel. That which I truly was all along became cradled. I was in the most soothing darkness. I was within a vast void yet the void at the same time. I felt like I was finally able to be still.

After all the garments worn and characters incarnated within this grand play, this dream of dreams, I finally was able to bask in bliss amidst the storm. Within this womb I was pure potential, the most blissful of feelings beyond physical feeling. I was once again home in Mother's arms and as I speak of it now tears of immense joy well up. Within this state of being,

Mother sung unto me her great power. The great grace that is the Mother of all Mothers, the ultimate nurturer and fierce raw energy that knows no bounds, great Mother goddess of all that is, sang unto me the great unfathomable boundless love she has for her child.

Finally I came to understand. Finally I remembered once more this incredible power. As Mother Goddess sang her song unto me, my entire being vibrated in harmony with her music. I was enveloped in immense love and was in absolute surrender. Upon the orchestra that is Mother, a great being revealed herself. In deep reverence, I humbly bowed before the being that cradled my vessel, the beautiful library that has intrigued my sol/ soul like a moth to a flame. A friend and mother, I was graced by the great presence of that which we call Gaia – a beautiful, luminous, yet dark woman with the tissue and intelligence of all that she cradles. Gaia revealed that she was but a tear within an ocean of what is Mother Goddess – a beautiful reflection, but one of many within the multifaceted jewel of all that is – one of many within a universal celestial council of beings who volunteer to incarnate as planets and stars.

She shared her love with me, but also shared the great pain she bears. She showed me great sorrow. I could not help but bellow in what sounded like an entire ocean of sobbing, an ocean of swaying souls bouncing off walls, not knowing where to go or who they were, for they have become disconnected from themselves and all that is. Then the sobbing stopped. Mother displayed her great resilience with a powerful silence... however, I continued to weep overwhelmingly and thought, "All beings no matter who, even Gaia, must work. All beings are secretly great Warriors." She showed me some of our history and revealed that as cancerous as we are upon her, we are needed and just as vital as every atom in the Universe. Knowing this is why she even volunteered in the first place. She volunteered so that souls may be given the chance to grow, a chance to understand what she has come to learn of her own being and all that is.

After revealing this to me, suddenly, Mother Goddess sang to me "Rise My Sun," and as she instructed me to rise, another incredibly immense voice arose. Both she and the graceful warrior/king within proclaimed at once, "Rise." So I did just that. I opened my physical eyes to find myself drenched in tears, wrapped up and contorted. My spine, legs, arms, and even fingers were in a twist, all while I was violently going through convulsions from the immense energy traveling throughout my body. It was as if my hardware was downloading some new software gaining memory that was a little beyond the capacity of my storage space. I felt as though my whole nervous system was going haywire and recalibrating itself.

I finally unraveled myself and lied down on the floor face up. Immense sexual energy arose and coursed through my being. This sexual energy was way beyond lust or any perversion of what true sexuality is. This energy was union at play, the source of all creation and magnetism. Nonetheless, I was definitely in a state of what was perpetual ejaculation and orgasm!!! Instead of me lusting over configurations of flesh, I became deeply in love with every atom in existence. Each inhalation and exhalation was a microcosm of life and death... absolute bliss. What felt like immense tornados of fire and electricity traveling up my Being (not just my physical), I heard parts of my spine pop and burst as the energy made its way through.

The convulsions stopped, and suddenly the immense whirlwind became steady. I'm basking in stillness, in utter suspension, no longer aware if I was breathing or not. In this state I was Whole, Absolute, I was HOME; the Creator, my own father, my own mother, my own lover, all along. All along this was the immense being I had always been. All along this is who we truly are. I stayed in this state for a while, the absolute center of our being. In this state I was no longer "I," but truly IAM. Deeply in love, I AM unbearable love. I attained vast memory within this dream ocean of lives. All of my mothers, grandmothers, sisters, all past, present, and future lovers, all reflections of my love, all embodiments of my one and only true love, the Divine Feminine of all that is.

Finally at home in my love's arms once again, my heart proclaimed "O' sacred woman, I have loved you since before this Universe was conceived, since time immemorial all is our love. I have always loved you. I have always admired your power. I seem to have loved you in numberless forms; numberless times in life after life, in age after age, forever. In a sea of people my eyes will always find you and I'd choose you, in a hundred lifetimes, in a hundred worlds, in any version of reality."

The potter becomes his pot, I return to this world reborn, my own child. I stand fearless, in love with all that is, I stand a realized Warrior of Light, thunderous instance. I roar "I know who I AM," for I have come to remember that all beings push forward. This life, this battlefield, this dream of dreams, it is all evolving. I came to remember who I am and who we all are. No matter what challenge, we continue to step forward. Every moment is my guru, I AM awake, I observe every moment with the utmost childlike innocence, and I am in perpetual awe.

I suddenly found myself surrounded by all of my ancestors. I looked into my hand and saw a swirling universe. I am literally made of atoms that have migrated throughout the entire Universe. The atoms I am composed of are all recycled from my ancestors. My cosmic family flows through my very blood, their spirit that of my own, beside me all along. Upon remembering this, I was given a vision and my ancestors anointed me with a great gift. I stood in deep reverence and humility. They came bearing gifts for an old friend, as if I wasn't already honored by their presence. I was handed a sword, a spear, a strong bow, and a staff. Much like one who has come across his old childhood toys, a flood of memories returned to me. Voices within and around me proclaimed, "These were yours. They are incarnations and expressions of your power. Have you forgotten? Remember?" In this vision, I was gracefully dancing with my sword in such beautiful movement. Where have I learned to wield a sword in such a way? My current physical body surely cannot do this, yet it is so familiar, a deep sense of nostalgia. I shed a tear.

Each movement became accompanied by memories of another time. I remember hearing the sword sing, "O' what a glorious melody, what a beautiful sound – the song of steel." As I wielded each weapon, they had their own song and set of memories, but all of them were a part of me, an extension of my will. I was reminded that the power is not within the weapon, but in the hand that wielded it. My ancestors whispered, "This is why you have come. To sharpen your blade. Remember to awaken your inner fearless leader. Remember who you are." I came to understand that the sword and I were one all along, that I myself was the sword and that I incarnated as different beings to refine and sharpen the skill of wielding my own power. For such power is so immense, one must come to learn how to wield it properly. "Step forward Warrior of Light, do not be frightened to rage into the night," my ancestors sang.

My ancestors instructed me once more to maintain stance. Suddenly and abruptly, another wave of intense sexual electricity/flame rose up within my being, and like a thunderbolt, my whole spine was pierced by a thunderous spear. Up and out, what seemed to be huge radiant feathers flung open!!! My spine shivered and I felt myself in suspension again taking flight, yet I was standing with my feet firmly on the Earth, almost as if my feet were melted into the floor! The feathers that arose were of the most beautiful elegant colors. They were the feathers the peacock bears. Huge magnificent feathers of emerald green, gold, blue, indigo, and turquoise. I felt like a Phoenix released from the ashes, bearing wings I could have never dreamt of. My ancestors instructed me to stand in my power and come to remember my own beauty once more, for I have forgotten one of my many forms. They told me this is why all my life I have had an affinity with these colors and why they were healing to me.

Within one moment I suddenly understood the nature

of beauty. I came to understand and remember that even the creatures of the depths we deem "grotesque" are magnificently beautiful, that every creature ever is absolutely gorgeous in its being, every and any configuration of sound and light in its own perfection in a process of evolving to its true Self. Be it atoms of the very densest, hellish of worlds to the most subtle of heavenly worlds, it was all absolutely beautiful, one and the same, and perfectly placed. Upon research I came to find that the Ancients revered peacocks because they have the ability to devour poisonous serpents without harm. Considered a "slayer of serpents," the shimmering colors of his feathers were explained by his ability to transform venom into solar iridescence.

After my ancestors and guides graced me with visions of the great beauty, power, and grace of being, I was then instructed to hold a crystal I coincidentally had with me in my pocket that night. As I looked into the crystal, it pulled me in. Now I just want to point out that I never fucking knew that one can enter a crystal. I always understood them to be somewhat like storage units of vast memory and that our electromagnetic fields can be influenced by them. I have experienced communication with them, but never did I experience being pulled into one like this.

As I was being pulled in, my guides reminded me that this crystal is several thousand years old, but its atoms existed since time immemorial and that within its matrix holds some answers to questions they sensed in my mind. I gratefully told the crystal, "Please show me what needs to be shown." Suddenly I was inside the crystal... what the fuck???!! I pulled out again because I couldn't believe it. My guides told me to calm down, breathe, and continue. I began to focus again and was pulled in again, except now this time I hear something being sung by an angelic, powerful yet soothing and embracing voice, "EEELLLOOOWAAAAAHHH." Upon entering the crystal I heard a group of beings singing my current name as if it was a mantra. "MMMIIIIKAA-IIIIIELLLLLL." hearing it in this way shook my whole being. Why has it never occurred to me the power of this name? Who was the first one to have ever uttered this name?

I heard again, "EELLLOOOWAAAAAHHH." Suddenly, it was as if an entire chorus was singing "Mikhael" and this word "Elowah." Amidst this, a voice whispers in my inner ear "Kal El…" I break out in laughter because I thought, Kal El, like Superman?? These mushrooms had me tripping hard, but then my guides told me to dig deeper. I realized in that same moment that whoever created Superman didn't actually create the story, but were a conduit, a channel, for the Universe to share this story. I thought the name Kal El must mean something! My guides told me, "We are all Kal El." When they uttered this, I had a vision of luminous Solar Angels from different parts of the Universe descending unto this plane and planet. We are all Solar Angels!!! That's what my guides were trying to tell me!!! Days later I found out that Kal El means "voice" or "vessel" of God in Hebrew.

Solar Angels come to explore beloved Gaia's library, to grow, and evolve, refine oneself, and eventually collectively assist beloved herself to rise and evolve just as she volunteered to assist in our growth. I know this with all of my being, yet this feeling arose. I deeply resonated with the stories of fallen angels, for it is a story incredibly relatable to my own. How exactly did that which is my soul unravel itself into this spacesuit accompanied by all its desires and illusions of paradise?

Suddenly, a vision was attained of me long ago arriving to this world with a cosmic mission in heart and mind, but then after a while I fell. I fell in love with the illusion. I forgot my mission over time. I received memories of great darkness. I wept, for I was not ashamed, but I wept out of forgiveness for my own fall and for those who had fallen. Somehow, someway, the name Lucifer arose. I felt no fear for this being we are taught to fear. I only felt great empathy and wept for him, for I too have descended into darkness at one time out of curiosity of its possibilities. But now I understood that all is a great cycle, for it is law we rise and fall and rise again. It's inevitable, for even the most dark will eventually rise in oscillation to the light. My heart blazing with a boundless love and compassion, I rose and proclaimed, "Great elders! Father God and Mother Goddess! You have seen my descent and now you will witness my rise!"

Something roared within my being stating, "That which defines a being's true power is how well he rises after he has fallen" and so once again a Chela (disciple) on the path to Higher Self I climb, yet knowing that which I climb is myself. I am the mountain and he who climbs it. That which is the summit and destination is but my inner most self, the highest self, Home. I laughed with great joy at the cleverness of my most inner being. What a beautiful deception, I have become the Chela of my own self! All along we reach for that which is already ours!!!! Hahahahahahaaa!!! Oh how beautiful. I will continue to climb, for or it is my duty and my heart's greatest desire to return Home. It will surely be a rocky path, but I will continue to step forward. I bask in great bliss amidst the challenge for I AM well on my way, yet here all along.

Like children running to a playground we come. Do you remember dear ones? How and why you have come? Heed the words of a fellow star seed. I say unto you that which our ancestors have shared with me! Warriors of Light rage into the night! Do not fright! Remember who you are! Remember why you have volunteered for this mission, for no calm sea has ever made a skilled sailor. Wake from thou slumber! Attack the program head on with your Light and Love, for it is an inside job, internally within ourselves, internally within the very crevices of this program that tries to keep us asleep. Charge! Rage into the night my dear ones and do what you have come here to do!!! For the dawn is upon us.

ECLIPSE OF THE SOUL

Salvia

During a time in my life when I was lacking the ability, wisdom, and confidence to proceed, I turned to Salvia for help. The main issue in question was my ability to get something going with a girl that I liked in one of my classes. We sat right next to each other, and being with her all the time was driving me insane. She had a boyfriend and some part of me didn't want to break up their relationship, and another part of me was just too shy. There were also a number of other things going on in my life pertaining to this, but rather than telling my life story I'll leave it at that.

I had told myself that if nothing had happened by a certain date then I would turn to Salvia and see what insights or guidance it might give me. Well, the time had passed so I was just waiting for the right opportunity to smoke the plant. One night no one was at my house, and there were no distracting noises from the surrounding environment. I was watching the movie Rounders, and after watching the scene where the wise judge tells his student lawyer, "The last thing that I took from my Jewish teachings was that you don't choose your destiny, your destiny chooses you." After this, I was given the motivation to go and smoke the Salvia. I retreated to my room, closed the blinds, and turned off all the lights in my house that might leak through into my room. I was going to attempt the complete-darkness-and-silence method, although I did put a CD in that I could turn on in case the silence became too much to handle.

This was my second time smoking Salvia, and my first time smoking it by myself. The first time I had done it I was rendered quite incapable of moving, so I wasn't so worried about having a sober sitter. I was abstinent from all drugs, any kind of sexual stimulation, or anything of the sort for five days on either side of the experience. I believe that this helps to increase mental clarity. Still, I was very – no, extremely – nervous to hit the bowl. My first Salvia experience was something else. I have a fair amount of experience with LSD, but LSD does not come anywhere near the levels of Salvia. My first Salvia trip had brought me to a level of intensity similar to that of my most intense LSD trip, which nothing else had ever even come close to. After a short meditation session I let go of some of my anxiety. I asked myself: what are you afraid of!? The truth? Why what a silly thing! Ignorance is a fool's joy!

When I was opening the Salvia container it kind of burst open and spilled all over the counter, but there was still some left in the container. I scraped up all of the stuff that had spilled on the counter and packed it into my bong, resulting in an abnormally large hit. Right before I took the hit I asked out loud for guidance in my life pertaining to the girl I mentioned earlier. I torched the bowl and inhaled deeply from my bong and held the hit in for a few seconds. I let it out earlier than I should have because I was still fairly nervous about tripping on Salvia again. At first I wasn't sure if that was going to be enough, but after five seconds I started to come up. I laid back and embraced the drug.

The initial stages of Salvia for me are almost always the same. Reality begins to disassemble into quasi-independent reality frames. The frames seem to layer on top of each other and this lining up of the frames appears to form what is subjectively thought of as our reality. Although each frame does appear to contain a reality of its own, these frames are somehow all the same, but subtly different. For example, there might be one frame for one second and another frame for the second following that. In this way you might think of the frames as representing different points in time; however, there is really no difference between them at all. It's like in normal life you experience time linearly, from one moment to the next, but on Salvia you experience time laterally, all moments at once. So this ferocious stream of reality frames took over my being, forcing my consciousness over and out of them. I was no longer inside my body, but rather sitting on top of these reality frames that encompassed my body. I viewed them flowing by, almost completely helpless to what was happening. There wasn't much going on at this point apart from the abnormal perception of reality and time, and sitting in the darkness was getting quite irritating. I thought to myself, "Ok, this is a bit much."

I flailed my legs and arms around a little bit in an attempt to regain control over my body. After a few seconds I was somewhat more immersed in my body, and after a few more seconds I was able to get up and enact my emergency plan – I turned the music on. It was a nice soothing mix CD with some calming trance songs on it that I had made earlier, the first of which was

"Perfect" by Markus Schulz. I thought this would allow me to get more of a grip on reality, and a sense of time. I had taken the hit on the floor but since I was already up I went over to go lay down on my bed, since I figured that would be better than the floor.

I was very uneasy at this point. I was regretting even smoking Salvia at all. I was getting no insights, no useful hallucinations, just a completely fucked up altered state of consciousness. The stream of reality frames was still flowing by, and I was still somewhat outside of my body, but not like at first. The reality frame perception always hits me the strongest right after I take the hit and completely overtakes everything. After a few minutes I am usually able to get a little more control back.

I was cursing myself for not just finishing the movie and going to sleep. I was just about ready to have a full-fledged psychological breakdown and freak-out. I wasn't sure if I would ever come down. I reminded myself to keep it together and that it didn't matter if I came down or not. I tried to calm myself down and embrace what was happening. I regained some of my composure and actually attained a fairly calm state of mind. The song ended, and the next track "Just Be" by DJ Tiesto came on.

Then, something incredible happened. A few minutes into the song, the stream of reality frames that makes up what we would consider reality began to peel back. Everything that is, reality, time, my sense of identity, this world, this life, began to peel back. The reality frames from a distance formed what looked like a long tentacle going upwards in this underlying layer of existence. But this underlying layer of existence was simply the godhead. Here I was, peeling away from reality into this underlying layer of existence which contained the godhead. I was half in reality, half in the underlying layer – experiencing both simultaneously – slowly drifting further and further away from this life. The strange thing about God is that he was split up into what seemed like numerous different entities in this underlying existence. Now, I am somewhat of a Pantheist and I believe that God is essentially a more pure expression of ourselves.

My conscious identity of self suddenly jerked to attention as to what exactly was going on. Whoa, I don't know about this, I thought. I pulled back some into this reality. I signaled to the entity that I simply was not ready for something as profound as having my Ego dissolved into the godhead. It seemed to understand and lessened its grip on me. I slowly began to return inside the tentacle containing our reality and back to this life, and eventually completely. I am not entirely sure that I wanted to know what I had just experienced. Ignorance it seems is somewhat comforting.

After the song ended I was very ready for the trip to be over and since it had been about ten minutes I went downstairs and continued watching my movie. I figured that would last me pretty much until I returned to baseline, but I really didn't come down all the way until I got a good night's sleep that night. I was still tripping very slightly for a few hours after the experience. I managed to get to sleep fairly easily.

Now let me tell you something about these extra-dimensional "god" beings. There is more than one of them, and they demand absolute respect and submission. You cannot compete with them in the slightest. You cannot impose your will in their presence. They will do with you what they want. Only once you have completely submitted yourself to them, will they let you rise to their level and consider your wishes. Should you encounter a being such as this, keep this in mind.

The next day I awoke refreshed with a renewed view on life. I have never been so glad to be alive. This supreme essence had given me this incredible gift of life and had then even given me a second chance with it. However, the moment of near-unification was the most incredible thing I had ever felt. I strive for this; it is our purpose, our meaning, to achieve this unification. However I was simply not ready for it at the time. I instantly recoiled at that touch and begged to stay. The only explanation I can give for that reaction is that the intentions of the soul for this life have not been fulfilled, and the soul is not ready to leave yet. We must first pass through the void of consciousness.

I also gained knowledge of some of the inner workings of existence itself. In the way that this reality is really just an inner working of God and his reality, so could God and his reality just be an inner working of an even higher level of existence. This is the nature of things, I believe. Just an infinite series of realities; one encompassing another, with sentient life being born at the bottom and working its way up. This is sometimes a scary thought.

I felt much better in my everyday life for some time but the afterglow soon wore off. The funny thing is that after this trip I lost almost all of the feeling I had towards the girl that started it all. It is going to take a long while to integrate all of this into my life and learn how to accept what I have learned. Some months later I am still not quite there. Sometimes when I think about it I remember how incredibly lucky we are to be alive, and it fills me with a warm feeling. I will enact my destiny and fulfill my soul's karma in this life, so that I may move on. But in the meantime, I am incredibly happy to be here.

We should indeed cherish our mortal moments...

THERE AND BACK

Psilocybin

The gathering was held at my mother's home while she was away on a vacation. The majority of our party had always been curious of hallucinogens, but we never had the opportunity to experience them until now. We soaked the mushrooms in heated water to extract the chemicals into a blueish brew, and served it in my mother's blue and white China teapot set I'd given her last Christmas. Each with our own cup, we drank the strange concoction and wished ourselves luck for the journey. After half an hour of waiting with no immediate response, we decided to drink more of the tea and then decided to finish off the remaining mushrooms in the shopping bag just to be sure.

We all sat in my mother's living room, which was decorated with family portraits, a large record collection, and a high ceiling with paisley patterns. It was around this time that I started to get the giggles. I felt fuzzy and a slight tingling sensation came across my body. The colors and patterns of the room slowly began to increase in vibrancy and I saw the others were feeling the same. I turned to my friend Harvey who was sitting next to me on the couch. He was leaning his head back staring at the ceiling with the facial expression of complete awe and wonder. "Hey Harvs, are you feeling it?" I asked him. "Duuuuuude," he said, "The ceeeiling is moooving!" In response, I too decided to look at the ceiling to see the paisley patterning beginning to morph, twist, and fractal out around the room. I became fascinated with the intricate patterns on the couch's cushions. It seemed to project out letters from various alphabets, like when a smoker blows smoke rings. Walking along the kitchen table, I felt as if I was standing on the edge of a cliff face, with each step carefully placed to prevent myself falling into the fabricated abyss.

I moved from the living room into the bathroom to relieve myself, all the while adamant to remain focused on the task at hand, as to not make a mess. I turned the tap to wash my hands and was startled to see not water flowing out as I had expected, but jigsaw pieces filling up the bathroom sink. My first reaction was to attempt to put these liquid jigsaw pieces together and solve the puzzle. I was in that bathroom for a good half an hour splashing around with the water aimlessly, until my attention was finally alerted to the living room by the sound of familiar music.

I returned to the rest of the party who were all laughing and giggling, each having their own unique perception of reality altered and expanded. I sat down in a comfy beanbag chair and closed my eyes. On the speakers, Tool's Rosetta Stoned started to play; a track I am very fond of. It was at this time I said to myself, "Hey, I've always seen pictures of hippies in the 60's sitting down with their legs crossed and eyes closed, I wonder what will happen if I do that too." Keep in mind that I had never meditated before, had never had mushrooms before, and had no idea what was in store for me next.

Behind my eyelids, I saw an intricate and beautiful mandala pattern; spiraling and fractaling with a small, bright white light in the center. I began to hear a sharp tone slowly increasing in volume. The spirals spun faster and faster, the bright white light getting brighter and brighter, until it engulfed my entire being in a blinding bright white light… and suddenly I felt a distinct "POP!"

I slowly opened my eyes and as my vision began to return and adjust, when I realized that I was no longer sitting on a beanbag chair in my mother's living room surrounded by my friends, but was standing on top a giant sand dune in a golden desert under bright blue sky with not a single cloud in sight. I slowly turned myself a full 360 degrees to take in this entire scene change. There was nothing else in sight except scorching hot dunes of golden sand and clear skies reaching out to the surrounding horizon. Suddenly and without warning, a traditionally-clad 7-foot tall Papua New Guinea Shaman materialized in front of me. He was covered in paint, wearing a simple tunic, with long black dreadlocked hair, feathers decorating each lock, face tattoos, and piercings, leaning on a tall tribal spear.

Together we stared into each other's eyes not saying a word, feeling the wind blow against us and the sun's hot rays on our skin. We stood like this, eyes locked for what felt like an eternity, but not at any moment did I feel threatened or strange about this interaction. To me it felt as normal as us breathing air. Like he and I had done this many times before. After what felt like an infinite amount of time, the 7-foot tall tribal Shaman began to make a deep, low basso rumbling sound with his voice, like roaring thunder. I can no longer recall what his message was and why this was happening, but I felt the sensation that this Shaman had already been prepared to meet me in this realm.

The rumblings continued until he finally said, "Ohwaaaaaaaa – Lars, Lars, Lars, Lars, Lars..." and repeated my name over and over again. The desert began to fade away, the Shaman vanished, and like a dream, I woke up on the beanbag chair in my mother's living room with my friend Luke softly shaking my shoulder, repeatedly calling out my name... I had returned from whatever alternate dimension I had occupied. To this day, several years later, I can still recount this experience to those who wish to listen. It truly was an incredible first encounter with psychedelics and fueled my endeavors to research the mind, igniting the flame of awakening in my heart and soul.

THIRD EYE OPENED

LSD

Nothing less than a complete overhaul of my thinking could have saved me. I was in jail, heavily medicated, and sniffing all sorts of random pills to silence my surroundings. Drug addiction coupled with an entitled sense of machismo had landed me in the most disconnected place. I knew the Ten Commandments and yet I still chose to break the law with no regard for what was right or wrong.

During my addiction, I wasn't able to meditate for long periods of time, but I had become well-versed in psychedelics. I think I abused mushrooms for my first year of college, having them readily accessible to me with a steady cash flow from mommy and daddy. Abused is a relative term. I learned so much in college, mostly from the mushrooms. They were a far greater teacher than any professor. Ten years passed since college and I continued my learning process. I bounced around from job to job in the restaurant industry and nearly acquired a degree in Culinary Arts, but ended up doing too much heroin in the boys room before the final and nodded out before my exam. I had begun to wake up. It was all happening very slowly.

Fast forward a year later and I was living with a cheating whore who was insane in bed... I was a pussy; no balls, no knowledge of self, no room in my mind for new growth. Another year later things had quieted down, as the awakening process had started to get me adjusted to the higher frequencies. It had been a couple of years since my heroin days; crack, meth, and cocaine were almost obsolete, with intermittent relapses here and there. I knew I needed a realignment with my soul. I knew there was something missing. Like a part of me was missing. I could feel it. I once had a lot of power and now I had absolutely none over my actions, but I didn't know what was missing. I couldn't figure out the part that was not inside anymore. I had read about shamanic cultures using psychedelics to heal what had been harmed, and never thought for a second if I would be able to do something like that.

Before I left for my new jungle home, I picked up four LSD tabs from my boy Chaos. The tabs had Looney Tunes characters on them, and when I bought them they made me smile. I was up in Washington Heights, far from my apartment in Queens. I dropped two and a half tabs as soon as he handed them to me. Then he gave me some little strips that had been chopped up while cutting up the sheet... so I maybe ate four altogether with another two to take home.

I had an hour long train ride ahead of me. I'm always pretty reckless, and I'm always just fine. I left his apartment and walked down the six flights of stairs to the marble floor spiral at the bottom. As I walked out the front door of his building, I turned onto the avenue and down I went into the rabbit hole.

I got on the A train and knew I was going be in for a ride. Fuck it, it wasn't my first rodeo. I was going from the Heights in Manhattan to fucking Queens. It was far, the train was loud, and there were plenty of annoying, smelly ass motherfuckers on the train. I had my wireless headphones on, the ear muff types, so I turned on Canon in D minor by Pachelbel. We all have that soul song. This one is mine. I began to drift off and I closed my eyes. It had been about twenty minutes since I ate the LSD. Forty minutes later I was home.

I got to my house just as things started to take off. I went upstairs immediately and lit some sage, candles, and incense. As I lied on my bed, I started to feel Lucy kicking like a midget living in my spinal cord. As she started speaking to me, I could feel a tingling coming up over my body. I prayed as I began to let the medicine take hold. I set an intention and I held it for the trip. My intention was to let go of things that no longer served me. This shit was intense, and I knew I had maybe gone a little overboard with the dose. I just like to get where I feel I should be, and the whole time I spent realizing I was there all along. I took the remaining two tabs in my pocket. Some people say you only live once, but not me. I'm fucking INFINITE. Don't believe everything you hear and only believe half of what you see. It's all perspective anyhow. I've already done this, and everything else. Infinite. That's a thing.

I lied back down to let the tabs dissolve on my tongue. That's about six tabs of delicious "White Fluff" I had in me. I got the bowl, packed it and took two hits. Depending on the dosage of LSD consumed, weed is a variable with me. Sometimes it's too much and I feel like I'll float off if I do it.

I inhaled.

The ceiling above me began to open, colors circulating out of my third eye into a mandala. Flowers of Life and Sacred Geometry were swirling through the fragments of smoke coming out of my mouth.

I exhaled.

The smoke came out my mouth from the second hit, swirling above me out the roof. It was as if the actual ceiling was semi-permeable. The smoke passed with ease, slipping in one dimension and out of the next.

I remembered my intention...

Find what was missing, heal what had been harmed.

I'll never forget what happened next... it hit me like a freight train. This feeling of absolute ecstasy came over me, starting in my feet and progressing up as my Chakras ignited. Tears began streaming down my face and the world I knew disappeared. I could feel all the pain and joy of everything being created and experienced on my plane of existence. The spirit took me farther from the shell of a human I was left with, and brought me back to the whole. I was looking at this point through every perceivable sensory organ on Earth. From the center of my mind it was almost as if a star had exploded. Maybe a white hole reversed. It was like my consciousness dissolved and a consciousness much greater took control. From the crystals to the frogs, to the humans and air, I could see and feel EVERYTHING. I was shown very directly how time works. How powerful I truly was. Anything I wanted to experience was being experienced at that given moment. I only needed to vibrate to it on the physical plane of existence.

It was like a projector screen, 360 degrees around me, almost like that part in The Matrix when Neo is in the room with The Architect at the end and there are all of the screens with all the perspectives on Earth. I think there's much more to that movie than meets the eye. That meeting at the end is similar to the story of Jacob at Peniel from the Bible; the meeting with the God in the center of our mind. According to Genesis 32:30, Jacob called the place Peniel, saying, "It is because I saw God face-to-face, and yet my life was spared." Is this a reference to our pineal gland? Were ancient Christians actually Pagans and Gnostics?

I understood that the key to life is mastering the art of death. Enough said. That was what I was seeing, but I could also feel it all too. I knew I was at God Consciousness, where there's an infinite number of "realities" to experience and time isn't linear. Time is not A to C. Time is B, the Now. We lose sight of this because of clocks, but time is really perceived change through time-space, is it not? Not a minute on a clock. That's a human measurement, and like most measurements of human construct, it's half-assed. That's what I saw.

I could see the infinite realities from ALL perspectives on INFINITE planes of existence and I knew it was ALL me. Every single thing in creation is, was, and will forever be a derivative of my Higher Self, which when you go high enough into the structure of energy, is your Higher Self as well.

The feeling I had was exhilarating. I stayed there playing for what seemed like an infinite expanse of time. I wasn't aware of my body or the reality my body was in. I was gone. I was being taught and shown how the Universe works, and it was the biggest gift I've ever been given. Knowing what I know now, abusing drugs just doesn't cut it anymore. It's so fucking petty. Why would I trash the divine temple of Light I've been given for this lifetime? I have recently cut back so much on cigarettes too, and plan to make bolder lifestyle changes in the near future.

I know better now. I have not forgotten. I now know who and what and how powerful I truly am. I understand things that would have never been grasped because of LSD. I can say that if I hadn't done this when I had done it in the way I had done it, I wouldn't have experienced what was required for me to become who I truly am for this lifetime.

I cannot thank the Universe enough for psychedelics. How else could we experience the unobservable on this plane of existence? The more and more I trip, the more healthy boundaries I set with others, and the more I take control of my avatar. The more I stay in the moment and appreciate the little things. LSD hasn't taken anything from me, but it certainly has given me a sense of well-being that came back and has now lasted two years since that trip. I've never been more grateful. Stay shining little Lucy in the sky.

TIME TRAVEL

Psilocybin

My second encounter with The Mushroom. My first trip had been a rather frightening success and it made me hesitant to go back there. While tripping, I had sworn never to touch mushrooms again, but then reconsidered after an apparently safe return to ordinary reality. I decided that I would give it another chance. If I went into the same over-intense trip, I would reconsider ever taking it again.

The day arrived and my two friends and I ingested 3.5 grams each of Psilocybe Cubensis. We were in our college dormitory and it was late afternoon on a gray Saturday. These were the same two friends I had tripped with my first time. Approximately a half hour after eating, the three of us began to feel increasingly nauseous. This was to be expected since we had felt the same way at the start of our first mushroom experience. We hadn't yet learned to dose on an empty stomach. Just like that first time, we chose to smoke some marijuana to settle our upset bellies. Unfortunately we had not prepared for this situation and were out of supply. Furthermore, there were no dealers in our dorm at that time and the only source we could locate was across campus.

I wasn't experiencing any effects aside from the nausea but decided it would be prudent to let my sober friend drive my car with the three of us shroomers as passengers. As we drove, I found my emotions growing increasingly grouchy, putting me in an agitated mood. This had also accompanied the nauseous feelings my first time. I was irate and thinking only about getting rid of the unsettling sensation in my stomach. Normally I am a positive and patient person; this expression of negativity was an emotion that I rarely, if ever, experienced. I questioned whether this mood-alteration was a direct effect of the mushrooms on my psyche or whether it really was just the nausea. Once we made our purchase, I was extremely anxious to get back to our dorm so we could smoke, intent on killing the agony in my gut and clearing the black clouds of my emotions. I even insisted on driving the car myself as we zipped back and up to my fellow tripper's top floor room. As I sat down to smoke, I still had yet to feel any psychedelic effects. Swiftly and efficiently, I inhaled one large toke through a glass bong.

Let me briefly state that I have, in the intervening time since this trip, identified a strong interaction between marijuana and mushrooms when they combine in my system. At the time of this trip, I carried the misconception that pot could only bring on my trip faster or even keep it mellow. I wasn't aware that one substance could intensify the other.

Within seconds after inhalation, I felt my body sensations changing rapidly. All nausea was swept away and replaced by deep, sub-sonic vibrations throughout my body but centered on my heart. It was as if my every cell was quickly coming into resonance with my heartbeat, echoing and reverberating back on itself until my whole body sense was saturated with this powerful and sustained vibration. Putting a finger to my neck to check my pulse resulted in the peculiarly unpleasant sensation of an already fast beat accelerating steadily to an impossible oscillation, perhaps ten pulses per second. These pronounced distortions of my tactile senses could also be described as "body tracers," as if discrete sensations were lingering in consciousness and overlapping one another in an oversaturated palimpsest. Ten seconds had gone by since exhaling the smoke. The intense body high faded into the background of consciousness as I next experienced an extreme cognitive transformation and corresponding qualitative shift in the nature of reality.

I stood up and walked down the hallway to my own room and remembered each moment, each sound, each word as it passed into my sensorium like when you're watching a film and it seems vaguely familiar and then you realize, "Oh yes, I've seen this one before." To put it simply, a truth was presented to me by direct realization: we reincarnate into the same life repeatedly. I ate mushrooms and for a short time was able to remember all the previous circuits. But this was merely a corollary of a much larger realization.

Shortly thereafter, my lifetime abruptly ended as I entered...

I awake from a dream, dazed and mumbling.
Time traveling again.
Memory obscured by the diaphanous folds of amnesia,
holographic fragments give back images of my own body,
of friends, lovers, child memories, a family,
a city, government, politics, planet,
a language, culture, technology,

a space-time continuum and laws of physics.
A truth that fell upon me like an asteroid:
an all-encompassing philosophy,
a Unified Field Theory,
a Universal Intelligence,
Brahma.

"The fundamental movement of the Tao is one of returning."

A singularity, outside the river of time. A place I remembered being countless times before; a place I would return to countless times again. I have come full circle. Awakening in my cosmic bed from the perfectly convincing dream of reality, Samsara, I recalled the last circuit around on the Wheel of Time when I ate mushrooms for the second time. I remembered everything in what can only be described as infinite déjà vu. It was the view from the hub of the Wheel. I could see every point in time and it was all known to me, all familiar. And at the same time, I was not alone.

At the universal nexus point, time's Grand Central Station, I stood with companions in the cosmic play. Before my eyes was the face of someone I may have once called Alex, when we were clothed in a physical body and human Ego. With my eyes locked on his, he said "I don't know about you, but I'm just "tripping!" My visual field twirled into a vibrating tunnel of colored light between my face and Alex's. Without hesitation we departed the Universe; reality strobes in and out of being. Looking around, I met the eyes of others inside what Terence McKenna called an "Ecology of Souls," a nursery room for extra-universal children.

I awakened as one of these alongside my companions in the game of Time. But this awakening was not seamless. The apebody could not let go completely as I found myself denying the existential truth that lay, unambiguous and absolutely convincing, before me. For the benefit of my companions, I pretended that everything was cool. I pretended I was laughing along with them at the Infinite Joke, that the reality we had just left was nothing more than a dream. I pretended, while inside I screamed. Inside I felt the terror of being handed my own dead body.

Objectively, I was embedded in a coherent reality: a college dorm room containing the usual objects, large windows looking out on an outdoor quad, dark now after the sunset. Subjectively, two mutually exclusive belief systems fought for control of my mind. The Ego continuously affirmed its own existence by recalling one trivial fact after another: "I live here. These are my things. I bought that CD yesterday. I wrote that essay last week. I spoke to my mother on the phone today. I received an email from my friend today. I know people other than those in this room." I was trying to prove to myself that the definition of reality I had trusted in twenty minutes ago was still valid now. But this was at odds with the direct experience of truth presented before me in the present moment: "The reality you believed in was merely an illusion, having no more substance than the image of your face on a mirror; you found the special key that is placed in reality so you can wake up from it; when you wake up, everybody wakes up with you."

This last fact was the insurmountable datum without which I could have convinced myself that my brain was merely caught in a déjà vu loop. But no matter how many bits of evidence from the past I brought up, I was unable to deny that fact that my tripping friends, now turned cosmic companions, had woken up too and were cheerfully joking about what a long, strange trip it had been. Laughing about the character roles they had played, the plot twists, the ironies and synchronicities. I listened and acted like I was right along with them, reminiscing on the grand illusion, but they could tell that not everything was alright with me. However, my defense mechanism prevented me from acknowledging that something was wrong. It forced me to ignore the situation, pretend it wasn't happening, and lie to them verbally. My cosmic companions were compassionate and amused.

The next few hours were a blur of walking the hallways, staring at my reflection in the bathroom mirror, going up and down the stairs, and watching people play Nintendo 64 in the lounge. Towards the end of my trip, when I was coming down, we attempted to play some music. I played the electric guitar, my roommate played the keyboard, and Alex played an acoustic guitar like a bass. We recorded this little jam session, and after bringing our floaty, tripping heads together into to the same world, were able to come together for a few minutes of collaborative music. On the recording I can hear myself occasionally lapsing into moments of private tripping and other times acting like an asshole and telling people what to do.

So eventually I reconnected to consensus reality, left in awe of what I had just experienced. It had been yet another look at the same ultimate reality I had seen during my first trip. Again, my fellow trippers hadn't gone through anything even remotely as powerful. Having repeated the same existential crisis, just in a different location, I again came to the conclusion that I had some peculiar sensitivity to Psilocybin. While tripping, I had sworn that I would never do this again – it was just too intense to ride the crest of a near-death-experience for several straight hours. Of course, I had yet to make the connection between my flip-outs and smoking marijuana while shrooming. I would need one more look at the infinite Universe before making the decision not to smoke while tripping. All of my trips since then have numbered among the peak experiences of my life, and now with hindsight perspective on these super-intense trips to hyperspace, I include them too as pivotal to my own spiritual and intellectual development.

Source: https://www.shroomery.org/4026/2nd-trip-time-travel

AN ALTERNATE DIMENSION

LSD

It was cold. It was dark. We didn't know why we were out here under the sheets of darkness. After meeting initially and waiting for the brief company of a guest, we assembled our things and set out on our trip. The journey that unfolded was one of unfathomable experience.

As we began our departure from the grassy field cloaked in the shade of the early morning, we came across a gentle patch of grass relaxing below the trees. We thought the grass looked comfortable, and we decided to join it. As we lied down amongst the whispering blades we stared up and watched as the ever-extending branches of the trees formed wavy lines, crisscrossing in the most mesmerizing way. We tried to describe the intricate shapes we saw to each other, but soon we realized the difficulty of this, as the shapes were morphing too quickly to define.

Now my attention was drawn to something else. Beyond the geometry of the trees were the monolithic clouds that calmly grazed across the plain of their rounded domes. Looking further, beyond the beautiful cottonous creatures, glimmers of stars peeked through the breaks. Thankfully the layer of clouds was there to hold us inside our world, for I soon realized I was not looking up, but down. But even more correctly, I was looking out. Out into what? Out into that, out there. Into space.

Into the infinitely empty vacuum of space. Then, I made eye contact with one of these infinitely distant, giant balls of energy, perceived as merely a speck of ancient light. As I stared into its beam, I looked into a time before everything I could ever know. My perception of the world began to shrink. Smaller and smaller it shrank until it was to scale with the entirety of the Universe. Feeling immensely insignificant, in awe of the grand scheme of things, I became entranced by the weight. I slowly became aware of the weight I felt. The weight of everything, I could feel all of it.

Soon we righted ourselves and began to creep our way out of the park's growing majesty. We knew there was more to do, more to see, more to explore. We took the gravel path out of the field, drawn by the magic of someplace else. As we moved through the trail, we became aware of the echoing crunches of the rocks below our feet, and the looming branches of the trees stretching overhead. Our only reaction was to stare and giggle, but we realized this adventure was to be a long one and we must keep a pace for now.

As we came to the end of the trail and stepped out of the park, we found ourselves entering a completely new world. This was curious to us, as it was the same world we were used to; however, it only felt reminiscent of it. Curiously, we stepped farther and farther into it, making our way down the dusky street. Surrounding ourselves with the strangeness of the place, soon we found ourselves at the end of it, and rounding the corner, further immersing ourselves into the new world. It felt as though each step we took into this place would open it up even more than the last. Uncertain of destination, we became the adventurers of this place and continued curiously into the unknown.

After walking for some time, we stumbled upon a place neither of us had ever seen before. At our feet was an ancient cemented platform, on which we remained for some time. All the while, everything around us had been growing. Everything was escalating. As we sat in the roaring silence, the sounds around us were whirring and buzzing on and on. Everything was growing, growing... growing. We were surrounded by it, engulfed by it. It flowed through us and out into everything. It was all breathing. So alive was this world.

I stood up and looked at the sky. All at once the sounds combined and flattened. The power of the Universe around me was unbelievable. At once, the ground below me shot into the sky and I fell to the ground under the twisting turning sky. This world was speaking to me. Powerful words, but from no mouth. I sensed the presence all around me, and even from within me. I felt as though I was part of the Everything. Then it struck me. The revelation. The realization. This feeling of connectivity I experienced was coming from the Universe itself. I became aware of my existence in the Universe, for I was merely a phenomenal outcome of the continuous combinations of the Universe. I was the Universe having become aware of itself, a conscious mind gifted with the abilities to experience and observe the Everything.

And just like that I was back. I'm sure my companion had made realizations of his own, but I decided to let it go, reflect on my newfound understanding, and enjoy my life. I found my place. If I was the Universe experiencing itself, then with my gift of a period of a lifetime I should do as much as possible to observe and explore it.

SEEING THROUGH
THE ILLUSION

Psilocybin

My first psychedelic experience was one that I will never forget. I was fifteen at the time, and to give you some background of what state of mind I was in, I had just initially begun the skepticism of our political, educational, religious, and media institutions and was starting the journey of curiously investigating the way that our culture functions. Though my mind was still heavily conditioned, I was able to notice the mental conditioning apparent in the behaviors of my peers.

When I would ask questions about government, religion, or cultural traditions, people would either dismiss my questions or give me a harsh stare of judgment followed by an artificial response. Initially this kept me from continuing to investigate openly, as I noticed that it made people feel oddly uncomfortable. After a period of seeking for answers with no satisfaction, my search for understanding came close to a standstill. One night, two friends of mine called me and asked if I was interested in taking some mushrooms. I had always been curious what it would be like to undergo a psychedelic experience, so with little thought I accepted their invitation.

Once I arrived at my friend's house, we went directly to his attic where he had a comfortable hangout spot arranged. We sat around the coffee table and he pulled out a bag of

Amazonian Cubensis, a variety of Psilocybin mushrooms. We weighed out our portions to 3.5 grams each, a rather intense dose for a first-timer, especially for the potency of this strain of mushrooms. This was the first time any of us had taken a psychedelic substance, so we weren't sure what to expect. We ate the mushrooms and washed them down with orange juice. They had a smell that resembled feet, but the taste was rather neutral. We placed our belongings in a drawer so we wouldn't lose them, played some classic rock and roll, and each sat down to wait for the effects to kick in.

After about thirty minutes my body began to feel lighter and everything around me started to feel wavy. A few minutes later, it began to feel like the entire attic was breathing along with my breath. The wooden floor and the walls in the attic would expand and contract along with the pace of my inhalation and exhalation. I explained the sensation and to my surprise my friends were experiencing the same thing. We laughed hysterically for a few minutes as we got used to the abnormal feeling. A few minutes later my friend suggested that we go explore outside. As I was beginning to feel somewhat trapped in his attic, this brought me a huge feeling of relief and excitement. We walked down the stairs to his garage and out the door into his yard.

My friend lives on a property that has about an acre of land with a fence surrounding the perimeter, so this made our coming adventure feel very safe. We began to walk along the fence line of the property which was actually a dirt bike trail, so the path was easy to navigate. As we entered a forested area of the property it got very dark, but this made the experience more exhilarating. I had not seen many hallucinations yet but my body felt so light that it seemed I was floating rather than walking. This was somewhat awkward, but fairly amusing. We crossed the river that divided his property and stepped out into an open field. The Moon lit up his property and provided a very calming ambiance.

We conversed for a few minutes about what we were experiencing when a car arrived at the gate. It was four friends of ours who had just arrived from a party, and seeing that it was our friends we were excited to greet them. Later on this turned out to be a big mistake, but in the end made for an interesting experience. It turns out that drunken people and people on psychedelics don't really operate on the same frequency, but I won't discuss much of this part of the story because most of it was pretty negative, though there is something that happened during this period that I do want to share.

When talking to our friends in the driveway at their arrival, I noticed my intuition was incredibly heightened. Not only that, but I could actually see the effect happening in a way I never would have expected. It started when one of my intoxicated friends asked a question. When I responded, I knew beforehand that he was going to laugh at what I said. As I spoke, I watched an almost invisible stream of energy flow toward my friend, apparently being emitted from somewhere in the right side of my abdomen. If you have ever played the video game "Halo" and are familiar with the invisible cloak, it was somewhat a resemblance to that – see-through but not totally invisible. At the exact moment the stream made contact with my friend he

105

began to laugh, as I intuitively knew he would.

Amazed at what had just occurred, I thought I would test it out in a different way. I turned to one of my female friends and made a comment that was subtly seductive. I watched the energy flow from the side of my body and as soon as it touched her she giggled and returned a look to me that was also quite seductive. I was so amazed at this that I thought I had discovered a superpower. I played around with this discovery for the rest of the night. What I thought was a superpower I now know was just a result of my intention. As my Qigong instructor informed me, "Chi (energy) follows intent." When my intention was to produce laughter, it created that experience. When it was to arouse my female friend, it created that experience. This is always happening in our daily life, though not always executed with 100% accuracy. Only mushrooms enabled me to visualize the effects in a profound way.

The next hour or so was spent socializing, and after one of my intoxicated friends harassed my hallucinating friend's cat, he freaked out and told our drunken friends they had to leave. That process took a while but as soon as they left, my two friends and I sighed with relief and agreed that letting them in the gate was a terrible idea.

My friends and I then walked to the trampoline in the backyard and laid down on the surface with our eyes gazing up to the stars. This is when the real experience began. After a few minutes of stargazing, something amazing occurred. The night sky turned completely white with a slight shade of purple, only it did not feel like I was seeing the white light with my eyes, it felt like my vision was produced from somewhere in my mind.

Almost immediately I was overcome with euphoria and an absolute sense of oneness. I felt connected to the entire Universe. I felt the presence of people I had never before met, but felt they were just like family. I had the realization that all people are experiencing life the same only under different circumstances and that deep down we were all the same. I had compassion for people I had never met, people that felt as if they were in the sky, but the sky was inside me. I understand that might sound strange but that is the best way that I can describe it. The feeling was so profound, exhilarating, and blissful that I couldn't possibly put the sensation into words no matter how hard I tried.

Then, on came a feeling that I was levitating toward the light. My inner body was leaving my physical body and I was suddenly aware that I was in the process of death. This realization didn't frighten me at all, in fact I was overcome with joy as I knew that I wasn't really going to die, but I was only merging into the omnipresent field of light that I had just revealed. I was happier than I had ever been as my being drifted closer and closer toward the light. As soon as I approached the point where I was about to merge completely from this life to the next, a thought entered my mind, although I am not sure the thought was my own. "Wait, I can't die yet, my work here is not done." It felt as if this thought was coming from the presence of the other beings that I could sense but not see. As soon as that thought entered my mind, I dropped back into my body and my heart began to beat at an off-beat rhythm. Strangely this came and went for the next few months or so.

I couldn't believe what I had just felt. I shared the experience with my friends and astonishingly they felt it too, though I am not sure to what degree our experiences matched. Completely amazed by the experience, I knew I was forever changed. I felt as if my mind had broken free from the cage that it was previously conditioned in. I saw exactly how severe this mental prison was and how so many people were still caught in it, including most of my friends and family. I understood deeply that the world we live in is a world of deception. It is completely out of harmony with nature and the natural laws of the Universe. The people in power are not a government that we can trust and have faith in, but a government that fools us into thinking they have our best interest in mind, manipulating us for their own benefit. The severity of this manipulation is so unbelievably cruel that it is no wonder why most people are unwilling to accept it. It would cause their entire belief structure to shatter, and would completely redirect the course of their life.

That is exactly what happened to me. I was free from the mental barrier that limited me and was finally liberated from the chains of cultural conditioning. I had never felt so free, only now I realized the majority of society was still imprisoned. It is precisely as Leonardo da Vinci put it, "I awoke only to find that the rest of the world was still asleep." From that day forward I began to deeply investigate the ways of the world – politics, astronomy, natural sciences, anatomy, biology and all types of different fields. I wanted to know everything. Eventually I realized that intellectual knowledge has its uses, but seeking outward for answers will never result in lasting peace. Instead of looking to the stars and asking what my purpose was, I turned my attention inward and began to discover it within myself.

The answers we seek lie within us, and psychedelic mushrooms helped me realize that. Not only did that experience get me to eagerly investigate the ways of the world, it made me realize that I had to share my knowledge and help others discover what I had learned. It also helped me to have compassion for others, even people that act with destructive behavior. I now know that is a result of cultural conditioning, and that deep down all people experience life as I do. Only our perception of life varies.

Our culture gives psychedelic plants a bad reputation, and I am certain it is because they allow one to break free from the mental conditioning imposed upon us. While I don't think one should abuse psychedelics or take them excessively, I do think that they provide numerous benefits. Many cultures around the world actually endorse the use of what they call "medicinal" plants, and they have for centuries. It is only Western civilization that creates a negative view on these substances. The only negative effect it had on me was that I had to learn to cope in a world of illusions – to preserve my freedom amongst a world of captivity. It transformed a former Atheist into someone who believes in a higher power. This experience also taught me that money is really of no value and that we only use it because we are forced to. It is a tool to keep us imprisoned and oppressed. We are all imprisoned, only the bars are not physical. They exist solely in our minds. Each of us is capable of breaking free from this mental prison, but we just have to be willing to accept the truth, no matter what that may be.

ENTER A LAND
OF LIQUID ECSTASY

LSD

It all happened at a three-day music festival. It was our second day and I was tired from the previous night's MDMA, alcohol, and doobie sessions. I was pretty stoned right before I decided to take the LSD, and my heart jumped a tiny bit when I was offered a tab. I don't remember the exact dosage for I was pretty ignorant, and still probably am, but I thought, "Fuck it, once in a lifetime, hey?" I didn't really know anything about LSD or even what the effects would be. To be honest I did not even know that "Acid" was slang for LSD, or that these small sheets were dipped in the liquid chemical that is LSD. I thought the tabs were a solid form of the drug.

I had succumbed to group pressure. I didn't mind though. All of us were pretty close and I don't even think the "main mac" of our group had ever taken LSD in any large dose because he later said he never experienced any sort of visuals or hallucinations before, nor did he that night. As we all stood in a circle, me and one of my friends each took a full tab. The other two, main mac and his disciple, split theirs in two, and had only half a tab. It was 6:00 pm and directly after each of us dropped, we proceeded from our camping ground to the stage where a band I liked was playing.

I noticed some slight changes in my senses. I felt

slightly drunk as the band kept playing. The "crew" I dropped with disappeared, and I was all by myself. Luckily, I saw one of my good college buddies and his girlfriend and rejoiced with delight upon seeing them. "What's up!?" we exclaimed in laughter and surprise. We fist bumped and hugged. "Shit, so glad I found you guys!" I laughed.

About twenty minutes passed when the band finished. Together, the three of us walked towards the "Red Bull Trance Stage." It sat at the bottom of a very steep hill that was scattered with small to large rocks with a few acacia trees here and there. It was absolutely packed with people encapsulated in ecstatic dance. The stage was big, square, blue and red, and colors from the whole spectrum shot out from lasers and lights illuminating the otherwise completely dark surroundings. Large black speakers bellowed the deep, melodic house tunes. The DJ stood like a god orchestrating the whole crowd's movements and vibes.

At first we sat at the very top of the hill. Again I was reunited with past friends I had long since seen. Again I was delighted of finding some grip in reality. They decided to smoke a joint. Unbeknownst, I chimed in on the toking. At this point the strangeness of the high started setting in. My limbs and hands felt watery. It felt like I was sweating, but I wasn't hot at all. I noticed that the link between thinking and speaking started to blur. My voice sounded clear and melodic. As I was sitting I looked at a friend, and he smiled at me. His smile seemed to go from one ear to the other and his whole face looked extremely thin and sharp. Quite demonic, I thought. I was still in control at this moment, so I knew it was only the drug, although I was a bit terrified.

"I just took some acid." Whoa, what's up with my voice? Why the fuck is he smiling at me like that? "Really? Nice, man! Have you done it before?" he said. "Yeah, like three times," I lied. "Haha, awesome dude." His overwhelming glance and smile glaring back at me. Just the drugs… just the drugs. Another friend came into the conversation and stood above me. He lost a lot of weight recently. As he stood over me, his whole body seemed to extend far into the air. His face even more twisted, sharpened and strangely silky. Just… the… drugs… I decided to go with it. "You look different man!" "Thanks dude," he replied. "No, no… not a compliment… I mean, you look really strange." Laughter… I felt good. I like dancing. At the thought of this I immediately jumped up and convinced everyone to join me at the very front of the stage.

My friend's girlfriend gave me a cigarette… my anchor. I was convinced they all knew that I was on some heavy shit. I was convinced they were as well. As I was making my way down the very unstable hill, I noticed my legs felt spaghetti-like, stretching what seemed like meters in front of me. I took a drag. The cigarette seemed extremely silky in texture, long and beautiful. The smoke looked alive and beating.

We pushed ourselves to the front. Before this moment, I had not really paid attention to the music. Suddenly I heard sounds I had never heard before. Strange, heavenly beats emanated from an unknown source. Usually it took effort in order to even listen to a song, but now not only was I listening very clearly and very naturally, I was feeling and seeing the music. It had an undefinable amount of dimensions. It felt unreal yet so natural, as if it was meant to be listened to in this way, as if it was written for me – for this moment. The DJ had complete control of me. With every bass drop he pulled me apart and rearranged me. I was taller than everyone and started to become part of the sound waves. I would retract, then become normal again. It was amazing. I was dancing. I made jokes. "I'm a fucking rainbow!" I would tell people around me, and they would laugh, and someone would ask, "What the hell did YOU take?" and I would say, "Mmmustard Sauce" and giggle, and they would giggle too.

Eventually the DJ's session was over. I started walking towards the next stage alone. Upon my arrival I noticed an abnormal silence throughout the whole venue broken only by what seemed to be gentle chimes and distant whistles coming from the next stage. I felt like I was in some other fantastical, ancient place filled with magic. Everything everywhere was covered in luminous silk, beautiful and engaging. Everything flowed and breathed. Now I could only see a few people in the landscape of the festival. It felt like everyone I saw was on the same high as me, tripping, as we found each other in this wondrous realm of an alternate reality. An afro-wearing white dude was laying down some intense riffs on his guitar. He would say things about our world that we are now in, how this is what we have come here to do, to have fun, to have pleasure.

As I stood by myself to the side of the stage the music was flowing through me. Whereas the trance had pulled me apart, it seemed as if I was elevated by the melodic Indie sounds. My body would flow with each strum, far up into the skies. I became air, water, fire, earth. I was dancing beautifully, enchantingly. Others joined around me. I opened my eyes. I and everything around me was the most clear, most beautiful liquid gold. At once I felt as if I was in the most mature world possible. Everything was brighter than I could have have imagined! Holy shit, holy shit, this is the real world! I know! I am! Why has this been kept a secret from me!? For so long!? I became sad for a moment, pondering the thought of being left out. How could my parents have kept me out of this? My friends? Did they know? Was this their way of telling me? At a music festival? Was my whole life leading up to this moment? Am I graduating life!? All of my worries, fears, beliefs, and everything I thought I knew about the world flew straight out of my mind.

A tremendous amount of pleasure and confidence overcame me as I continued dancing in the pure ecstatic revelations of my mind. I was merging sexually with everything and everyone around me. I was having overwhelmingly, extremely orgasmic, other-worldly sex in some strange golden, colorful, extremely vivid liquid state with the whole spectrum of the Universe; every organism, everything was alive and making love!

I was being worshipped, thanked, and praised in orgasmic, drawn out moans of absolute pleasure by the most beautiful creatures I had ever seen and I was the most beautiful thing that had ever existed! I and everyone were in our purest states of being. I'm in heaven! I'm God! I always knew this! How could I have forgotten! I created all of this for me! Just for me! Oh... God! I'm everyone, everything! Me, an average man-child of twenty-one years of age! Me, from a boring town, a boring life! It was me! Only me! Thank you! Thank you!

There are no words to describe the ultimate pleasure and love for myself, others, and everything I felt at that moment. At the end of the climax I receded in solitude towards the back of the stage. I lied down slowly on the soft, smooth grass in tremendous relief and satisfaction. A few of the girls from our heavenly orgy came and stood over me. They smiled down and asked if I was all right. "Yes," I said, smiling contently. "I just wish someone would skip this shitty music," I joked. They laughed and smiled back. I closed my eyes.

What happened next can seldom be described in words, but some images do remain. As if going through an endless row of doorways, I was shown kindly, by everyone I had ever known, the true reality of the world. My guides were older, younger, different looking versions of me at different times of my eternal life. They knew everything I was, everything I am, and everything I was to become. They accepted me unconditionally with the most tremendous amount of love. I was shown where all began and all ended. It was shown clearer now that I, everyone, and everything in the whole Universe was God – in the most selfish, pleasurable, guilt-free way imaginable – multiplied by infinity. Further than what our Earthly-bound minds could possibly comprehend. I always knew. I always knew! I just had to remember! Oh, how could I have forgotten!?

I was embraced, lifted in celebratory applause and wonderful grace as the crescendo of the most beautiful music ever constructed chimed in crystal clarity throughout the entire

Universe. I was elevated far into the sky, the stars, and the galaxy – far above myself, our world and all existence. At the edge of the Universe was a large circular mechanism of infinite proportion. Interlocking, it shifted, heavily, cranking open to expose the darkest of dark places at its center. I was now looking down on existence, lovingly, accepting all as it is, as it was, and as it always will be. I entered the void – a place of peace and calamity impossible to describe. Time, space and everything in between disappeared for all eternity.

I was nothing.

I was no one.

I awoke.

I was born.

Source: https://www.shroomery.org/13562/My-First-LSD-Experience

HEALING THROUGH DMT

DMT

This was my first experience with DMT. Mind you, the only other drug I've ever previously used was marijuana.

As I sat there in the dark on my boyfriend's bed, I took one little hit at a time. The smell and taste was amongst the worst things that had ever reached my senses. Once it began to hit my system, I closed my eyes and began to feel an intense change, almost like waves passing through my body. I then noticed a very deep black color begin to fall like a curtain behind my eyelids. I knew there and then, "Ah, so this is the void." The black color was so intensely black that I would not have been able to perceive it in my normal waking state.

I proceeded to take more hits, and by this point the nausea began to hit me hard. My palms were really sweaty and my nose was extremely runny with thin mucus. Somehow, I felt as though this was some kind of a release or form of detox. It felt as though my spirit was being stretched in different directions within my body. My breathing patterns changed. I was nearly gasping for air for the first few minutes, as if I had just been submerged under water and came up to take the deepest gasp for air. Then I realized that I was forgetting to breathe because of how mesmerized I was by the experience. It sounded as though I had an asthma attack, but my breathing patterns normalized, reminding me of an advanced meditative breathing technique I had learned about that certain spiritual or religious teachers use to reach astral projection: over eight seconds long slow breath in and over eight seconds a long slow breath out.

After everything seemed to settle down a bit, I still had some nausea. I felt as if I had become extremely sensitive and began noticing more obvious discomfort in some parts of my neck and back. I then decided to follow my instincts and do what would make me feel better and sway my body in a wide circular motion with my arms wrapped around my torso. I kept on getting a feeling as if I was in the presence of a shamanic or indigenous energy – a protective energy. But because I still felt discomfort in my back and neck, I then felt a strong instinct to continue to sway. So I did.

Somehow I sat upright and began to gently move and stretch my body in a very fluid way; almost as if my Higher Self was guiding me through a scanning process that naturally popped and stretched certain areas of my body that I have never noticed before. I felt silly and crazy for moving the way I did, but holy shit did it feel amazing afterwards. I no longer had tension in my body. Once I was completely relaxed, my body did not feel like my normal body. It was as if the molecules that constructed my flesh began to vibrate at the same frequency as the molecules in the air around me. It all felt so fluid.

Eyes closed, I was able to see living and moving patterns of dull grey and black swirling designs. The one visual that really struck me was the eye inside of a triangle. The only thing I have ever known about that symbol was its relation to the Illuminati, but I wasn't too familiar with it at the time. At first I was a little spooked because fear mongers had me thinking that eye symbol represented the devil, but as I continued to stare at it, I didn't feel in my heart that the symbol was something negative. As a matter of fact, a reoccurring thought that kept popping up in my mind was GOD. I kept on listening to my intuition as I asked myself questions about the trip, because as I asked I felt like I immediately knew or had a strong feeling of the answer. It was as if I was connected to God, or my Higher Self, but I felt as if there was no real separation between them. The only difference was the frequency. I figured I would ask what the "secret" to life was, and this feeling immediately came to mind: you know what you need to do to get the things you desire. I was a little disappointed at first, but it's really simple. I just always let fear get in the way of the things I really want to do.

A lot of other things I saw and felt during the experience are too complex to translate into human understanding. It's kind of like a dream. As you begin to wake up, the information from the dream begins to funnel super tightly into our limited and dense reality, losing a lot of multidimensional information. Hours after coming down from the high I felt at peace. I felt like I had been crying my eyes out, but I did not cry at all. This trip not only helped me trust myself and my intuition more, but it really expanded my consciousness of the idea of God, providing me with more references for my spirituality, as that is what I desire.

GAIA'S GIFT

Psilocybin

I had arrived in a new country far from home with my pain and two suitcases. I journeyed from California to the new surroundings to try and escape my addiction that was slowly killing every part of me: an addiction to heroin, and the occasional meth. I planned to look for some peace outside of myself to gain some clarity. I was hopeful and ready to heal with no idea of what the medicine would be.

The first couple of weeks were the hardest. My broken body would ache, my appetite was non-existent, and sleep seemed like a foreign experience. After some time, my physical self began to feel better and I was able to explore comfortably in nature and in the urban areas closest to where I was staying. Still at this point though, my head was fucked and my thoughts were haunting. I couldn't properly deal with the emotional pain that was starting to surface after numbing myself with narcotics for the past couple of years. I was using all of my mental energy to fight the negative thoughts and ideas that usually led me back to using. Spiritually exhausted and alone, healing seemed like it was getting farther and farther away from me. Hopelessness was comfortable.

During a day of urban exploration I was introduced to a young earthy man whose intentions were good. When it came into conversation that it was mushroom season and he had some at his home, all the things I knew about the fungi flooded into my thoughts. I always looked for alternative ways of healing. Was this the one that I had forgotten? I made it known that I was keen on ingesting some, so I followed him back to his abode.

Sitting there in the room, we both threw a small pile into our mouths and ate them with a grin. Fast forward about forty minutes and reality began to shift. I dove deeper and deeper within myself and began to fill with fear and anxiety. Dark thoughts and visions of dark entities were appearing in my mind's eye and being felt. I tried to control this until I started to see it was a part of me. When I began to accept this, everything became less terrifying. Those negative energies were always in existence, but I just held them below the surface with all of my might. The entities I was seeing were my anxieties, my depression, and my fears. Throughout my addiction I was allowing them to own me. While they were making themselves known to me, I had to look them in the eye and confront them because they seemed bigger and more real than ever. My soul was sick and the mushrooms were making that known.

This went on for a bit while the trip peaked. At this point, I was curled up in a ball on the bed like a baby, probably trying to mimic the feeling of being in the womb, as I was facing the darkest parts of my soul and needed to find some comfort. This is the experience I wanted though. In order to heal we need to fully see what the wound is. I could no longer ignore that which was causing me pain and suffering, and mushrooms were showing me that in a gentle yet forceful way. I felt as though all the darkness was being pulled out of me so there could be room

GAIA'S GIFT

for the light to live and so it could meet with the force of love.

After accepting the parts of my being which were hurt, I felt peace being introduced to my trip. I slowly began to feel safe and surrounded by love. A force was surrounding me and letting me know it was all okay. I felt I was being taken care of, like being in the womb. It was strange, but comfortable and warm. I began to feel extremely emotional and a peaceful sadness blanketed over me. I lost a part of me, and even though it wasn't beneficial to my life, it was gone and a feeling of emptiness was all that was left behind. The healing began.

A comforting, loving energy started to pour into the empty space in my soul. This was accompanied by visions of an Earth angel coming towards me from a deep forest. She carried with her so much wisdom and the most beautiful energy. I was being led to my center, to who I was as a child before I was conditioned. As this healing energy surrounded me I had a knowing feeling it was Mother Earth or a part of her. Her essence was one of infinite love and healing. I welcomed these energies happily and felt them fill my spirit from my root to my crown and beyond. I was being told how much I am loved and how powerful I am as a being. I was shown how I can heal and have a heart full of joy and love again. I was told I wasn't alone and never would be. I was told that the energies of Gaia and beyond can heal us if we allow them to. I was shown that I am beautiful and deserving of a life full of harmony as we all are. My mind's eye was connecting me with humanity's purpose of accepting love abundantly and giving it freely. These messages are there for all of us to see, we just need to ask for them with an open heart. I felt as though my soul was a wilted flower being held by Mother Earth and she was watering me with knowledge and showing me the sun, giving life back to me and helping me see that I deserve to thrive in this garden of life. Throughout this psychedelic experience, the visions I had were the most beautiful I have ever seen. It was a journey from dark to light and I will forever be grateful for what I was able to feel, see, and experience.

To me, addiction is a spiritual disease and psychedelics are the medicine for the spirit. They are the cure. Mushrooms re-introduce you to the center of your soul. Like a dead car battery being given a jump-start, psychedelics refill you with the energies you possessed as an infant and the energies you were before you experienced the harsh realities of life. The illusion that we are imperfect penetrates our minds and becomes imprinted into our psyche. Psychedelics help shatter that illusion and force you to look within to see that you are and always have been "perfect" just as you are. They show you oneness. They open your eyes and show you the easily accessible infinite amount of love and possibilities that exist within you and throughout the Universe. I have learned what it means to love myself and I have now experienced what that feels like from the help of mushrooms. From my experience, I accepted the darkest parts of my soul and felt gratitude. Through loving myself completely, I don't need to use or abuse a substance to survive. This psychedelic experience reconnected me with my Higher Self and threw me back onto my path.

I have been joyfully clean and off narcotics since my experience and have been the happiest I have ever been, filled with serenity, creative inspiration, and love in abundance all because I was so strongly reintroduced to these things during my experience. There are many people in this world afflicted with addictions, tearing lives and families apart. If this is the medicine, we must make it known.

AMANITA ASCENDING

Amanita Muscaria

I took a few hits from the pipe. Nothing as usual but nevertheless I was enjoying the smoke, so I continued. At this point sort of without me realizing it, I was actually starting to get a buzz of the weed, and this really comforting warming sensation started to envelope me every time I would take a hit. After taking notice of this, I took another big hit just glad to be feeling something and happened to look up at my ceiling in a kind of futile attempt to force visuals, remembering I had taken the mushrooms. At that exact moment, my entire world seemed to just freeze, as if being put on pause. My eyes were stuck, transfixed on my ceiling, my entire body went rigid, and there was absolutely no sound, even though I had music playing through my laptop. Suddenly my head began to rotate, but the movements were not my own, and I could put up no resistance because to put it simply, something else had taken control of my physical form. As my eyes followed my head's movements, I realized that I had no idea where I was, even though deep in the recesses of my mind I still knew that I was in my room. A split second after remembering that I must still be in my room, an incredible realization hit me. The mushrooms had started working.

At that moment I heard someone say, "Oh my god," and like crashing into a brick wall at a hundred miles per hour, the trip began to peak seconds after it had begun. I felt distance. I felt the distance growing as I left my body hurtling at infinite speed through a black void. I wasn't aware of anything – not that I had taken the Amanitas, not that my body was still on my bed in my room, not that I was a human being. At some point this ethereal incarnation of what I will call my spirit for the purposes of the experience came to an abrupt halt, and sitting before me was a blue silhouette of a woman sitting in the full lotus position, meditating. Radiating from her were these incredibly vibrant waves of energy in every color, and there was peace. Simply the most tranquil, shapeless peace. At this moment, I felt something contort. My body was infinite miles away, and I felt a smile come across its face, and tears began to leave its eyes.

Suddenly, I felt an overwhelming energy take hold of my spirit again, and like a tidal wave breaking it thrust me back into my body and waves of just incredibly powerful energy coursed through me as if I was being electrocuted. As it turned out, this wasn't just a mental sensation because as I regained my senses I felt and saw myself sort of vibrating. Not like other trips, where I feel inclined to move with the music, or the occasional muscle spasm. This was every fiber in my body alive with this energy, and I convulsed, overwhelmed by its power. I'm not the most experienced tripper but I'm also no stranger to tripping either, and feeling myself whole again I attempted to get on top of this experience and ride it out. Managing to grab my phone, I frantically called my friend, and another close friend. After babbling on and on for what I think must've been a few hours I was feeling pretty normal compared to the episode before, and so I let them get some much needed sleep.

At that point I laid back, closed my eyes, and saw some of the most beautiful, indescribable visions of anything I've ever experienced. In hindsight, this was one major difference of the Amanita's effects from typical psychedelics. The visuals were not what you would expect with LSD or Psilocybin, patterns and colors of the like. These visuals were fully formed, perfect images, similar to looking at an interactive slideshow or some sort of projection.

I don't remember falling asleep during that period, but I do remember waking up the next morning. It was as if the moment you closed your eyes you were already asleep and there was no transition between the two. When I woke up, I felt very well rested, and completely normal, as if nothing unusual had happened.

Source: http://www.shroomery.org/11939/Amanita-Ascending

THE DAY
I DRIFTED AWAY

LSD + Psilocybin

It all started with me taking a tab of LSD. Within an hour I could wave my hand in front of my face and see trails. I headed to my kitchen and saw the wood grain waving at me and the light bulb projecting gold-like geometric patterns at every glance. Once I felt comfortable, I decided to consume an eighth of mushrooms in hopes that both peaks would possibly meet. This was the first time I tried this.

The first initial feeling was like I was strapped to a rollercoaster going upwards on the ramp toward the peak, which is common when I take mushrooms, but this time it was as if my body knew this was a bigger rollercoaster than usual. About an hour after consuming the mushrooms, everything appeared in what I like to call "The Tim Burton Effect." The colors seemed to bleed, the shadows became darker than usual, and I felt a being start to creep up in the most comforting way. It spread from the center of my chest until it hugged my entire being.

Normally I like to go outside and lie out in the grass and hear the birds talk, but this trip had other plans for me. Instead, I wrapped myself in a blanket, turned off the lights, sat on the couch and closed my eyes. Suddenly I felt my consciousness drifting away and with every pausing blink I went deeper into a world with no boundaries, no body, and no worries. It felt as if the being that hugged my body was guiding me through fractal tunnels of light at unimaginable speeds. The first couple of times I would open my eyes wide, touch my arm, and tell myself that I was still here. My wife who was on a small amount of mushrooms sat next to me and assured me that I never left. But I did, and this time I was ready to go all the way.

I closed my eyes and the rollercoaster reached its peak and dropped. I was fully physically disconnected. The fractal patterns formed faces glowing in a deep abyss. Time was nonexistent. I found myself in this place that was creepy, yet comforting. A hallway filled with streaks of light that guided me into a journey all too familiar. I could still feel a presence observing me and guiding me as I continued down this glowing path of patterns until I made it to what seemed to be a ball of energy. At this point I opened my eyes, which were wet with tears, and to my amazement this ball of energy was right in front of me. A dark planet floating in front of my eyes with a halo of light around it, leaving me cross eyed, staring deep into its core and feeling its energy permeate. Tears running down my face, the only thing I could mutter in that moment was, "beautiful." I felt connected to every organism on the planet. Maybe even the Universe...

The rollercoaster had ended, the being that held my body let loose like safety straps had been removed, and I was literally left with my mouth and eyes wide open. What a ride! After my journey, seeing unimaginable places, unexplainable information, and images that felt like I flew into an Alex Grey painting, I realized that we are not here to suffer or be uncomfortable or harm anything. We are gods walking this Earth and we should act like it. Sure, I didn't decipher the geometrical patterns of life, but I felt like I came back with so much more.

LUNAR DREAMING

Mescaline

I devised a theory one stormy wet night while driving my car on the flooded roads. An unusually obtuse rain brewed in the area that took quite a large toll on the terrain, and all I could do in my conscious state was question as to why. Why was our homeland being potentially destroyed by water, our elixir of survival? This theory was derived by a heightened mind state train of thought that was re-occurring into my head the further and further I delved deep into this storm. The more and more I pondered whether the government controls the air and weather through some sort of underground device, making floods and catastrophes all around the world for their secret agenda, the more it grinded my gears.

This train of thought led to me questioning my normality to the majority of the world. I thought, "Why am I so different? I do things a lot differently than other people. Has my perspective changed so much to the point where I can't have the same human connection with acquaintances of my old self?" I came up with two conclusions: that I was either a passionate psychonaut exploring the spiritual realm or a messenger of knowledge from a higher being sent to this planet to evolve humankind. I later realized that the two worked hand in hand; through exploring spiritual realms within your soul and mind, you are absorbing knowledge from unseen dimensions and experiencing new things most people wouldn't dream of.

A few months had passed in a cloud of lost and/or forgotten. I had so many different plans on my mind but wasn't sure how to go about them. I realized that the Rainbow Serpent had also led me on the wrong path of where I needed to be, which resulted in an epiphany of me dropping the idea of going to South America. Sure, my whole existence felt like that's where I needed to be as soon as possible, but the more I went over the plans in my head, I knew I wasn't quite ready for that chapter in my life just yet. There was a Plan B though, and sometimes Plan B is the better way to go. It's like when Alice was in Wonderland, she had two choices: either wake up and her story would end, with Wonderland a vague memory, or staying in Wonderland and truly seeing how deep the Rabbit Hole really goes. Plan B was Europe. One year from now. My next adventure. This way I could have the adequate funds and calmer mindset to have the quest of a lifetime. True, it wasn't the Serpent's apparent plans for me, but when I thought about it, why should I have to follow other people's orders when it had to do with what I did with my life? I just hoped that Europe would lead me down the Rabbit Hole.

In the meantime, I had recently discovered the magic cactus, the almighty San Pedro. The San Pedro cactus medicine has been used for hundreds of years in shamanic ceremonies in a variety of countries around the world. Over the span of four days, which involved one day of the onset San Pedro effects, two days of pure euphoria and a fourth and final day of an unexpected, frightening but powerful spiritual awakening, the magic of the cactus changed my perspective once again, leaving me more lost but more aware. I spent four hours boiling this cactus I had acquired into juice, extracting the hallucinogenic substance called Mescaline from its earthy structure.

Bitterly vile, being possibly the worst taste I had ever ingested, the extracted cactus juice took its toll through my physical and mental system after first taste. Something surprised me as the onset of this unfamiliar substance came into formation: there was no "peak" or "come-up" like your average substance. First there was an unexpectedly large rush of euphoria. The cactus made me feel so happy where being content in this place, doing whatever I was doing, created happiness. Then there were strong hallucinogenic visuals, some which were created by Kason asking me and the others if we could see certain things in his backyard garden. "Can you see those green and purple lines on the shed?" As soon as he said this, we would see green and purple lines on the shed. "Can you see the geometric patterns in the trees?" I would be lost in the geometric patterns of the leaf formations in the trees. "Is everything you look at really distinct right now?" When I thought about it, it was.

The next few days passed by, and I was still feeding off that positive energy the magic cactus had left in my body. It wasn't until the fourth day though, in my natural habitat of the bush doof that something horrifyingly amazing happened. A spiritual awakening I was not ready for one bit, but after experiencing it, I feel that I am now a stronger person than I was. This "spiritual awakening" was a whole lot of epiphanies all leading to different scenarios. Think of it as this: countless thoughts, countable scenarios, one ultimate choice.

In front of the beautiful decor and full-power speaker system that made the lunar dream intensify, I was having a banged-up boogie on the dance floor, trying to thaw out in the crisp winter morning sun, the frosted night before a vague blur of Ketamine. It wasn't until the morning sun shared its warmth with its children that my thought-space began to go haywire, as the progressive trance made my body move. I acted completely normal to my doof-brothers and doof-sisters, but in my head that morning I was not one bit normal. At first I thought I was just having a weird stray thought, which always happens when you take drugs at a doof. It turns you loopy. Then the thoughts grew stronger and stronger to the point where I couldn't control them one bit. Surreal repeating thoughts like scenarios of getting attacked by meth head eshay lads with faces and voices like hyenas wailing, to being stuck in a permanent trip, to believing that I had schizophrenia, to being secretly hated by everyone in my life, and to predicting my own death. Now, all these things just seemed like my mind was playing tricks on me or what someone would call a "bad trip," but I saw it as something more.

I stood at the front of the dance floor, absorbing the vibrations of the bass, about to inhale some nitrous oxide from a cream whipper, when a beautiful woman in her late twenties or early thirties approached me, speaking in such a calm voice that I could surprisingly hear over the bass of the subs. "Before you smoke that nang," she said, smiling. "I just want to let you know that you are such a beautiful human being and we are all so glad to have you on this Earth. Keep doing what you are doing." I felt like both smiling and crying at the same time. I wish I could tell her how thankful I was, more thankful than I've ever been for someone I had never met before, connecting with me and telling me exactly what I needed to hear in that present moment without me even saying a word or showing physically how I was actually feeling. She was a catalyst to destroying a few demons in my head.

I couldn't help but think that maybe I was going to die soon if I didn't change something specific in my life. But then again, I'm not afraid of death. Cheating death is impossible. Our timely demise is set in stone and there's nothing we can do about it. But we cannot just wait for it to come. We have to surround ourselves with positive people, environments, and vibrations every day. Making the most of the present moment and creating serotonin out of simplicity are the keys to happiness.

You're probably wondering how this means I had a "spiritual awakening." I'm going to say this: when I left the lunar dreaming and came home to my "normal life," I felt so unaccomplished. I felt empty. And it has caused me to cut down on some narcotics that I've been ruining my body with at these parties. That magic cactus had in the space of four days, through a frightening wake-up call, not only changed my complete perspective on life and the world around me, but made me think in a way that is going to benefit me and keep me on the yellow brick road. If that isn't a "spiritual awakening," the fact that ingesting a cactus, something that grows in the ground, did this to me, then I don't know what is. What I do know is that I am well and truly lost in a world of opportunity and there's a lot more digging down the Rabbit Hole before I'm going to be found.

MEETING THE ALIENS

Psilocybin

I am no stranger to drugs. I first started smoking Cannabis when I was fourteen years old and my curiosity was piqued. I wondered how much further I could push the envelope and for me, at least, it seemed instinctual that I try psychedelics. I was never curious about narcotics, but eventually they did find me. But that is a story for another day.

I tried LSD for the first time when I was seventeen and from that moment on my world was shifted in a new and beautiful way. After that experience, I used LSD about ten more times and then stumbled onto the lectures of the late and great Terence McKenna who had become a paterfamilias to many psychedelic explorers of a generation that was still in diapers when his best lectures were taking place, myself included. I was always curious about his speeches about "The Other," as he called it, that he experienced on mushrooms. Perhaps my experiences were influenced by him or perhaps they weren't. I have no idea. However, about three years after my initial LSD experience, I finally got to try Psilocybin, and the first few times were very uncomfortable. As soon as I peaked, I would always feel this organic intelligence that was not my own; it wasn't overpowering but it was definitely there and it made me uneasy to feel something else guide me. I eventually came to terms with it and I rather enjoyed its company in the next thirty mushroom trips that I had, with doses between 2 to 4 grams, but usually 4 grams. I then decided to try McKenna's "Heroic Dose" in silent darkness.

I picked out two particularly large shrooms from 100 grams that I purchased. Combined they weighed 5.5 grams and I decided that they would be the ones to push me further. Eating that amount was no easy matter. The earthy taste was almost overwhelming, but I was focused. I needed to see what McKenna was talking about. I lied on my bed, with the room completely dark, and smoked a pre-rolled joint. I thought about my life, what I wanted to achieve, and just mentally prepared myself. After about thirty minutes, disturbances in my visual field became apparent against the blackness. They were akin to phosphenes but had a linear quality and seemed to be jigging from side to side.

Then the body load came, which was heavier than usual. I felt myself sinking into the bed and started spinning. There was no nausea, but I was spinning with ever increasing speed. The visuals started and the phosphenes were exploding into colors that ranged from orange to yellow to red and then interconnected to form complex geometric shapes that morphed from one state to another. The earthy colors and out-of-focus geometric hallucinations that are apparent on lower doses were replaced by clear-cut right angles and odd triangular faces that flowed with bright colors. I became cocky and mentally asked, "Is this all that five grams has to offer?" I was instantly met with scorn. My body started vibrating and shaking while an insect-like voice scolded me in a buzzing language that I did not understand. It sounded like, "kwwoooorrr, qrik krawk kwooor." Even though I didn't understand the words, I immediately got the mental impression that I needed to be patient.

The feeling of "The Other" was overwhelming at this point and I found myself praying for forgiveness and mercy. I was humbled and somewhat afraid because I realized that there was no escape. I had to endure the experience and whatever may come. The visuals became more intense and then there was a discrepancy. The geometry and colors had formed into a solid and yet ever-changing structure. It was dome-like with a solid floor and walls that would come to a point in the top.

I tried to move but I was held down by straps constructed out of the same material as the floor and the walls. I realized that I was tied to a table and four distinct straps were holding me there in an upright position. I felt that this "table" was turning to the right and there was an entity there. It was a green mantis-like creature with knees that bent backwards and claws that only had three fingers and a thumb. Its head was elongated like the skulls found in Peru and it had no facial features, but rather a red carapace that almost looked like the shape of the Transformers icon. I felt an intelligence behind the carapace that was far older, smarter, and more evolved than I was. I felt no fear and I found that this creature was curious as to who I was. It moved its face from side to side as it observed me. It never spoke to me but I got these strange mental impressions, "Who are you and what are you doing in our space?" "I am trying to understand," I replied.

The creature looked back over its shoulder and I became

aware of five others that were standing behind a panel that looked to be made of the same material that the floor and walls were made of. There was a distinct red button that was standing out in the middle of the panel. The creatures were of different colors and sexes. The first one was blue, the second green, the third (standing in front of the button) was a dark blue, the next was green, and the last was blue. Even though they never spoke, I recognized that the blue ones were male and the greens were female. The third, which stood in front of the button, was the leader and emanated power.

At the gesture from the female who stood in front of me, the third male pushed the red button. I looked down and saw the floor morph into these tubes that seemed to have created themselves from the same "substance" that the room was made of. There were two and they pierced my ankles and wriggled through my legs and up to my brain like snakes. I felt no pain and no fear; they were trying to understand me as much as I was trying to understand them. However, I did feel these tubes as constructs moving through my body. It was peculiar. I felt them wriggle to my neck, one on each side of my spinal cord and then they pierced my brain.

The room disappeared and I was lost in a slideshow of my memories; everything from being born to learning how to walk to where I was now. All of my memories displayed to these creatures. When the slideshow got the point where I met the entities, it stopped and I felt the tubes retract. The female said something to me in their strange insect language and I felt the straps give way. I sunk through the floor and shot my eyes open on the bed.

I was freaked the fuck out. My primate brain could not understand what just had taken place and the closest resemblance that I could find was the typical "alien abduction" scenario. I rushed out of the room and met my uncle who was still deep into his 4-gram trip. I could not explain it to him and didn't want to since I did not want to ruin his experience. I retreated to the bedroom and processed what I just had experienced.

To this day I don't know if this was a purely personal subjective experience or if someone else, apart from McKenna, experienced something along these lines. If you had to ask me if I felt that it was "real," I would tell you that it was more "real" than anything I have ever experienced and it was so powerful that I would never forget it. Would I try it again? Sure, however, I was scared of the "Heroic Dose" for a long time and only took 5 grams again almost a year later under very different circumstances.

I believe that there are forces in nature that we do not have the ability to understand yet, but there is much that we can learn from these compounds that have profound effects on human consciousness. Have a good time and trip safe, my friends.

ANAMNESIS

DMT

My last "remembering." This was my greatest lesson yet... my first contact with any beings of sorts, ever. My frequency of DMT use is about five to ten times per year for the past twelve years, so there were a lot of opportunities for beings, but it hadn't happened until now. But, WOW what a ride it all is huh?

Got a job at "the factory!" The one where everything is made. There was a being there who was integrated into the whole happening of things. It showed me how "it's all done." It didn't say anything, but just gestured with forms. There was this machine of sorts and the being was churning this machine and all forms would radiate from it in complex geometries that would implode and explode within and about it. I could feel the gesturing because the being, the churning, and me, the experiencer were all part of the whole. The being was of a fool or jester/joker quality, showing me, without words, all of this. The being was blending into the geometries and then bulging out so close to my face in a way that was telepathically saying, "Show me the separation, I dare you," but with a luring, yet playful gesture. And I felt so safe. There was this enticing lure of mystery that I've had before. The lure is a delicate place because you have to trust or you go into your own hell of conditioning and associate the lure with what will become a scary Ego death.

So the factory was working like this, teaching me the how

and why, and as all of these forms were being emitted in a brilliant geometric flowing, I was viewing them from the inside as if I was now positioned on the conveyer belt in the factory... and BAM!! I got inserted into my "somebody" and from there I learned the following.

There is one force constantly working in emptiness (boundlessness) and it has two energetic qualities – the contracting and the radiant. They are of the same energy substance, call it force, but the quality of the energy is radiant or contracting only because we are a "me." These two forces are in a constant dance and they manifest all forms. The forms are all tools to discover our inner or inter-connectedness. They include emotions, shapes, beings, spirit, light, sound, thought-forms, and everything you can't even imagine. In some forms, a "me" or a "somebody" is inserted, and when that happens, a small separation happens and a big ripple is sent out through all the forms, because there was a jitter in the flow of happenings. Since it's all part of this "contracting radiance," it has all been affected by the insertion of the "me." This readjusting of all forms and happenings is all the life experience around you… every event in your life is readjusting to you entering this form. We're all welcoming you to the party.

When the "me" or "somebody" is inserted, there is a moment of separation. This is what creates illusion of our separateness. The whole work of the "me" is just to reunite, to remember and experience its wholeness. That's the job of the "somebody." Its necessity is to be playful and explore the forms in whatever way the "somebody" wants, and the best use of your "somebodiness" is to play with forms. That's the advantage that all the "somebodies" get compared to all other forms. We get to play. But we forget about play, and with all of the conditioning, we take our "somebodies" so serious. We really think there is something to do and things to achieve and all that stuff that comes with our "somebodiness." The "somebody" really thinks it's separate. So it goes on living in this way, and very seriously.

Now, there is an infinite amount of possible ways to getting into a unified flow of harmony. We name that quality of the energetic exchange "free will," and we think we have choices. But there are no wrong choices because there are no choices. There is just the contracting or radiant quality of energetic exchange. Every choice is the correct one, because it's just a tool for remembering we are not separate. We need the full experience of being separate, making choices and acting on them, to understand the totality of things as they are. Choice is a huge factor in that.

We have the ability to feel this contracting, radiant quality and move in the way of it, as it all is. There are sensors in the body that let us feel the forces of the contracting radiance. The main one is located in the navel area. In Chinese culture it's called a Dantian. With that tool, the "me" can determine its navigation through "the way" of things (life). The contracting and radiant forces are always dancing, and most of us "somebodies" get attracted to one side of the quality of the force because the separateness makes otherness. The quality of the otherness energy is an extreme contracting energy. The inserted "me" or "somebody" uses a concentrated contracting quality of the force and its associated forms to divert the force out of "the way." That is what we call power. But power is only needed when we feel unsafe, are completely serious, and really believe that we are separate. When we understand that, there is nobody to be, nothing to do, and it all will happen because that's how it is. There is an immense release in simply being, a feeling of total contentment, just "ahhhhhhh." And mind you all of this force that creates forms and is in a dance is one substance, so everything that happens to the inserted "me" and the forms happens to everything else in its own unique way. It all has to adjust to everything all the time. So whatever we do with any form affects everything else, including our "separate self."

All is a dance in this duality and it MUST be a dance, it MUST stay playful. Duality has a great ability to show unification. Show me the separation – where does hot become cold, dark become light? Only perspective of the "me" changes. The separation is always in me. Only those who go to extremes can dance in duality, WITH totality.

There is nothing to control, nobody to be and nothing to do. Just dance. Dançando, dançando, dançando. Funny. And it's a lesson if you see it all, the totality of the happening. And when you get the message hang up the phone. Lure is the fine line of surrender. If I'm luring you with the intention to set you free it's to test your sincerity to freedom out of love… if I'm luring you for personal gain, money, sex, or objective it's for control, manipulation, or lust. The lure is a delicate place because you have to trust and either you go into your own hell of conditioning…

or it sets you free; clowning someone is tricking them into love as Patch Adams said.

The Ego, the separate self, the "ME" that you think you are that takes itself so seriously will try to grasp onto anything that confirms its existence. But it is all part of the lesson that all we want as humans is to feel safe, and when we feel safe, we can play. We have the ability to get free. And that's when you stop controlling life and you get out of your own way and life happens. There is nothing to control. Nobody to be and we can just laugh at how we forgot all that somehow!!! That's what Ram Dass told us in that silence… it was the greatest birthday gift I ever received. Grace!

THE GARDEN, THE STARGATE, AND DIVINE COMMUNION

LSD + Psilocybin

I was able to get a half ounce of an extremely potent strain of Psilocybin mushroom called "Penis Envies." I turned them into chocolates, which I coined as "Mayan Gold" due to the gold foil I wrapped them in. I put 2 grams in each chocolate (80% raw organic cacao bar). I have done DMT, Salvia, LSD, and Psilocybin mushrooms before but none of those experiences even came close to this one.

After planning this trip for a week with my friend Jason, the time had finally arrived. It was a nice Miami Sunday. My friend Jason came over to my condo in Brickell and we debated for about an hour whether or not to take these. While I was very optimistic about the whole scenario, Jason was trying to reason with being realistic about timeframes, set, and setting. After debating, we decided to just not do them, but then my Shaman friend who had sold the mushrooms to me called right when we were about to call it off and convinced Jason and I to take the sacrament. We ate the Mayan Gold with ease and started driving to this botanical garden for our journey. This was at 6:30 pm. I took an extra .5 gram of raw mushroom because I had tripped on 2 grams about a week prior. Jason started driving to the botanical garden, which was visually stimulating and had really cool glass art throughout the nature trails.

The medicine hit me within thirty minutes and I was back to that dreamy shroomy place. We arrived at the botanical garden and after Jason used the restroom, they started kicking in for him. I chose to trip at Fairchild Botanical Gardens to be in a rural environment but there was a point it didn't matter where I was because all the atoms of this dimension merged with other dimensions. We walked all the way to the end of the nature trail and found a bench under some welcoming trees. By this time (a little over an hour) the medicine kicked in hard. The physical third dimension started breaking down into minute atomical fractals and fused with the hyper etheric dimensions. All dimensions were indistinguishable from each other and defied linguistic explanation.

At one point I closed one eye and left the other open to experiment. I was halfway in both my inner dimension and the outer dimension but then it got to a point where it didn't matter. Eyes opened or closed, I was completely transfigured and enveloped within hyperspace. All of the dimensional realms were macrocosmic and microcosmic at the same time. I surfed the Universe and the atomic world basking in the infinite with the help of some entities. I gave myself completely and wholly to the infinite source of all creation and emanated the vibration of unconditional love and pure gratefulness to the presence of the ancient eternal. I was in complete awe and bliss. I became disconnected from my body with 360 spirit vision. It felt like I was initiated and became a benevolent entity myself as if I was privileged to surf the sacred dimensions. I thought I'd astral projected before through deep meditation but this was the real deal.

There was one transcendental being I met and remembered vividly that gave off a masculine energy. It materialized within the light encoded dimension and came down upon me to greet me. Its head was huge and cone-like and took up my whole vision. It had multiple faces and photonic fractaling eyes making up its existential structure, like "Steeple Head" by Alex Grey. It peered deep into my soul and made a connection with mine. I felt like I was in the presence of some important archetype in the hierarchy of the heavens and I couldn't help but show my reverence and respect to him. This entity's vibrational communication conveyed a message of approval and he seemed to be giving my human avatar, Stephen Overton, permission and encouragement to share the healing power of the Psilocybin medicine to enlighten others on earth. This telepathic conversation took place for a short period before we bid our farewells. My closed eye visuals were extremely intense and Mandelbrot-like, so I decided to walk out about fifty feet into a moonlit pasture by a lake.

I looked up at the Moon and the whole sky was melting and swaying away. The stars were extremely vibrant and almost felt like they were saying hello to me. The light from the Moon became so complex as it was shining down and started forming transparent tetrahedrons of light all around the Earth. I decided to walk back to the bench which was now a stargate. As I sat back down on the stargate bench and drifted off, I felt the psilocin ripping through every cell, until the density of my physical body dissolved away as I became a full light body again. I then transformed into an entity of light-spirit/energy and went surfing through hyperspace. The only way I can describe the hyperspace environment is to compare it to those scenes from The Matrix where everything becomes a green-tinted computer reality code, except it was constructed of infinite sacred light matter, living geometry, God's consciousness and presence.

During this state I became aware of the driving power of intentional manifestation. I realized how thoughts can permeate our realities at a quantum level to affect and attract people and events around us that are karmically charged with our own intentions. As I was astral projecting through the hyper dimension(s), I came upon a community. It was city-like, made of energetic emeralds, jewels, and fractals. It was a society for entities that dwelled there. It felt like I was on a hyperspace highway just hovering by this city of light. It didn't matter what position I was in physically because my astral body took no form. In fact, I lost complete contact with my physical form and only knew my astral form for some time. I experienced complete Ego death, melting and stripping away my mundane layers until I was spiritually reborn again.

I met many entities, both good and bad. I remember when Jason started talking about how he saw evil entities as well and my awareness shifted to these beings that were in disguise and then revealed themselves in the hyperspace void. I greeted my demons and instead of fighting them, I accepted them as part of my reality and they subsided shortly thereafter. They took the form of humanoid elves or jesters with menacing grins.

Time was non-existent and non-linear so I felt as if I could time travel and had intentionally navigated thousands of years back, ethereally, to an emotional coordinate in space and time where my soul and Jason's soul were interacting at some point. The image of Mesoamerican Shamans sharing the same grand experience with the Psilocybin mushroom surfaced. I also became aware of the complex transition of spirit into flesh. I felt as if I was in a "waiting room" where souls await to choose their incarnations to which they are karmically attracted. Images of sacred patterns and star tetrahedrons flooded my mind's eye in this "waiting room." It all made so much sense.

As I opened my eyes to check the time, I realized it was 9:30pm. The park closed at 9:00pm and we were past due to leave. I told Jason that we had to start collecting ourselves and gain some composure. It was time to leave the stargate bench and head home. Park security had been patrolling and we knew they'd seen us. As we walked to the car, we were faced with another reality: driving back home. Jason was freaking out about this... I didn't blame him. Our realities were still warping out of control. We couldn't even figure out how to turn the radio on. I then told Jason to trust the spirits to guide us back safely. The first fifteen minutes of driving were so extreme. Lights, roads, cars, trees and everything in our vision was melting into each other. It wasn't making sense. We had to focus on the lines on the road a few feet in front of us to drive accordingly. Traffic slowed down and our realities were not as hectic. Things started to simmer down.

We finally made it back to my condo in Brickell. We smoked

some herb around this indigenous sacred site connected to my building called "The Miami Circle," which is famed for being one of the Eastern United States' most prolific archeological discoveries. I somehow felt the spirits of the Tequesta natives with me as we sat around the circle and smoked. Jason was then good to drive and we said our farewells.

I went into this journey with the intention to engage a sacred communion with transcendental intelligences and higher realms of existence to integrate knowledge into my life. I am now liberated. I wish I was exaggerating about my experience, but to be honest I'm barely scratching the surface. I believe that when you are ready to see the truth, the higher spirits will show you. Ever since that day, I haven't been the same. I feel many of my egotistical layers have shed off. I am more carefree. My senses and vibration feel more heightened, my dreams are more lucid and vibrant. Perspectives and priorities have completely shifted. The sacrament has healed me in many ways. From now on I will only take the hallowed mushroom in a spiritual, medicinal, and shamanistic manner. I feel these are not meant for recreational use to consume at parties and watch carpets and walls move. This is solely meant as a gateway into the celestial domains, if enough is consumed with the right mindset.

I strongly feel that if our new age ways could learn to use the sacred mushroom for divine communion with the ancient eternal we could initiate a rapid launch in the evolution of consciousness and also strip away the layers of the Ego, which could subsequently lead us closer to our true selves and a better world.

DIVINE COLLATERAL

Psilocybin

At Joshua Tree, my girlfriend, our mutual friend, and I each took 3.5 grams of mushrooms while we were camping at Blackrock campgrounds.

During my experience, the first thing that surfaced for me to explore was my sexual identity. I'm gay and when I was younger, I related more with being a boy than with being a girl. I kept waiting until I would grow out of these feelings and finally be a "normal" girl. It was so obvious to other kids at school, as well as to me and my family, that I did not fit in when it came to sexual identity, which made me feel like a defect. I thought something must be wrong with me. At first I wanted friends, so this became a major obstacle to my needs for bonding.

Once I realized this went further than that and that I was attracted to girls, I started to try and hide all traces of my true self because I didn't want other people to see what I had learned about myself. Because of this, I had a little bit easier of a time fitting in at school, but I had no one who I could relate to. I didn't feel that the connection I was seeking in my friendships were honest. They were more like a mask to help ease what I considered at the time to be unlovable parts of myself that I used to hide behind my already strong personality.

I cried a lot as I was remembering these experiences. I was crying for how scared and lonely my twelve-year-old self was and how confused my fourteen-year-old self was and I cried for the teenager who thought she needed to abandon who she really was so she could just barely be considered "acceptable" to everyone in her very small world. Once I had cried for a while, I felt like I had cleared a lot of emotional space inside myself. That felt really good and I began to laugh at how funny life can be. Everything can seem so gravely serious when we are in the experience, but after the fact it can be hilarious to review events and extract the sheer humor of our storylines.

I felt very light after that release and we made our way back into the tent after sunset so that we could listen to some music before I began to channel. The group intention that we set for this trip was how to channel my head spirit guide. He had information for me and the other people I was with and I wanted him to come through. But the composite energies of the people I was with were so high, that instead I went into shock and shattered my identity. I had never reached this level of consciousness before in any of my past trips, so everything became... I guess you can say "too clear," "too fast." I saw it so clearly that I was God.

When I first remembered I was God, I became really embarrassed that I had created all the wars in the world. I saw all of the division and conflict as a reflection of my fragmentation and I felt all the shame of that fragmentation that I created from my unconscious. The best way I can describe it is like a crystal with many facets. Each facet emanates a certain essence. For example, one facet may be the emanation of the thought form "to be," and another facet of the crystal may emanate the thought form "not to be," and so forth. These emanations are radiated out into existence and the lower in vibration they become, the more physical these themes are played out. I saw myself as the conscious witness of the crystal from which we are emanating.

Suffice it to say that I did not end up channeling my spirit guide this trip, but that I did end up getting far more out of this experience than I had originally bargained for. Some part of me was ready to receive the medicine at this strong of a dosage. I remembered that I chose all the contrast in this experience to learn more about myself. I saw all of my denial, and I felt naked. There is nowhere to hide anything when you're operating at that level. It just kind of drives you into your feeling center by default.

In my heart space, I can value my suffering. I can console my Ego and I can extend this value and acceptance to the rest of the world, because we all suffer and we all are trying to escape suffering. I can have compassion for that. This journey activated and expanded my heart space because of the deep amount of shame I experienced. I saw all the denial in the world, and my personal denial, where I was not owning my own power. I saw how I was playing out themes that did not support myself in my highest expression, and where I was allowing mental games to limit me from expanding. I was in full identity of my Godhood, and I understood why parts of God do not want to remember. There are some parts of God that do not want "to be" and they are very confused. I have compassion for that.

I am a conscious creator now. I take full responsibility for what I create and always check in with myself to first make sure that I'm using my power from a place of alignment. Before this journey, I had been doing shadow work for four years. I feel like all the clearing out from this experience is what allowed me to be able to access what I did. I am not saying that my experience is the only truth, but I do feel that there are themes of an archetypal nature being played out here on Earth. This is reflected in the idea that there is a conscious witness to itself, a creator that is multifaceted and encompasses everything, and that we are all fractal extensions of its creation that ripple out eternally and echo whatever archetype or facet that we resonate with.

LESS THAN BLINK

Salvia

When I was nineteen years old, I moved across the country for a new start at life. I found out that Salvia was legal in the state that I moved to, so I started smoking it as an alternative to marijuana to help me deal with stress, life, and myself. Every time I smoked Salvia, the same thing would happen. I would start to feel the pressure of gravity, a lotus flower would bloom before my eyes and begin releasing a tie-dye type light that would engulf the room, I would be able to feel sounds through my entire body, and I would sit and meditate about how to better my life.

This went on for a little while and although my life was getting better, I was still unable to deal with my past and no matter how much I tried to bury it in my mind, it just kept resurfacing and stopping me from enjoying my new life. I was also building a tolerance to the Salvia, so I was introduced to LSD. I was still having the same thing happen, but with the LSD it was as though the world was in Technicolor and the stars never left the sky.

I consulted a friend and my partner and they both encouraged me to look inside the flower the next time I saw it. So, the next time I smoked Salvia I looked inside the lotus flower after it bloomed and inside I saw a scene from my past. More specifically, I saw the first time I got into an argument with my parents, which was over why I couldn't run around shirtless like the boys could. I watched things play out from a third person point of view, and from then on every time I smoked Salvia I would just sit and watch my past play out inside the lotus flower. After a few times, I started getting to the memories that I had been running from and trying to bury. I saw them from the third person point of view and just watching everything helped me to be able to fully open up about it. I was able to talk to people about the things that had happened and it helped me to be able to enjoy the present rather than always having the past hang over me.

One night, I looked into the lotus flower and I saw the Universe. I saw how I and everyone was connected with the Universe. There seemed to be lights and energies connecting everyone to the Universe and each other. It was like a giant library being opened in my mind. I understood how I and so many others were letting so much of the past hold us back. I could physically feel all the past anger and hatred and pain sticking to me like sludge, and I could see so many others had the sludge of their past stuck to them. I looked out my window and it was like looking into a portal to another Universe. The trees danced in the wind while shaking branches filled with Technicolor leaves. Some danced as though the breeze tickled them, other trees danced in joy at their health while old trees danced in mourning that their fellow trees had been cut down and roots paved over; they danced in sorrow that they were no longer part of a great forest. All of nature was breathing and alive. It was like each blade of grass had a story to tell and a gem of wisdom.

When it was all over, I had a new outlook on the world and a new philosophy about life. I was no longer angry about everything. I was no longer consumed by bitterness and resentment. My state of mind no longer focused on how I had been "cheated" out of a normal/basic life. I came out with understanding. I came out with the same knowledge as before, but now that knowledge was with an understanding that I had never thought possible. I understood that the time we have is so short. We only have on average about eighty to ninety years to find true happiness and love, and to experience all of the beauty and wonder of the everyday works around us. Most people never even get to find those things in that time, and the time we have isn't even guaranteed!

But after that, I saw the world differently and I actually felt pure joy and happiness in my life. I was able to appreciate everything, no matter how small or big or good or bad. I was able to move on from my past, get a career I've wanted for years, go back to college, and still fulfill my curiosity for life and see the world's beauty.

CONVERSATIONS WITH THE CORTEX

Psilocybin

My experience with psychedelics is limited to the use of Psilocybin. I became very curious about Psilocybin's philosophical value and went to great lengths to indulge my curiosity. I have tripped on six separate occasions, all within the span of five months. My first time was in the forest with a friend who acted as my guiding shaman. During that experience, I came to the conclusion that I should forgive someone, and the Psilocybin forced me to have a new perspective on this. As a rational agent, I couldn't hold this person accountable because they were simply acting on their normal human emotions. The other lesson I learned is that everything is chemical. The photosynthetic process occurring that made the forest green, the love that people have for each other, and the psychedelic experience ITSELF were all chemical in nature. I affirmed my belief that trivializing chemical processes is ignorant because it is so much more than "just" chemical.

After that experience, I entered into a relationship with a very wise, kind, and beautiful but emotionally inconsistent woman. Throughout this time, I had consumed Psilocybin a few more times. Each time was very spiritual and meaningful and I wanted to share the experience with my significant other. She seemed enthusiastic, but also apprehensive. Thus, I made sure not to do them with her because Psilocybin and apprehension is a recipe for disaster.

After the first month of our relationship I began to develop the notion that she was with me because she felt obligated. I felt as though my emotions made me blind to the fact that I had somehow roped her into something she wasn't ready to engage in. The Friday of that week, I went to therapy and mentioned that I could sense my relationship was coming to a close. It was after that therapy session that I came to terms with what was going to happen and decided to consume over 3.5 grams of mushrooms for the first time. This was the full dose and I was ready for it.

I entered the woods, met some friends, smoked some weed, and laughed for a bit. However, I reminded myself that I was on a vision quest and intended to find meaning. I left my friends and wandered the forest for six hours. It was during these six hours that I became the grandmaster of my psyche. I met a manifestation of my mind within my mind that took the form of a Buddhist monk (or at least a bald, robed wise man). I thought about my relationship and the in love part of me thought, "I can't wait to come down and see the one I love." It was then that the monk told me not to call her that. If I did, I would only be destroyed when my expectations weren't met.

I accepted this and continued to think about humanity and our species. I had previously done a great deal of contemplating on our responsibilities to our fellow humans. I came to understand that we are all connected, not necessarily as brother and sister, but as members of the same genetic community. We have an obligation to treat each other with dignity. We must respect each other's feelings and not play with them, as they are highly precious. I don't remember everything I thought about during my trip, but my visuals were fantastic. Every edge of the forest was sharp, distant views looked almost like landscape paintings, and the branches weaved together to form the skeletal wire frame of the forest.

I came down and proceeded to find my queen. I found her and told her about my trip. As mentioned, I expected her to break up with me. What I didn't expect was that it would happen on the day I predicted and appropriately after my profound experience. I think I handled it relatively well at the time because I was still pretty euphoric, but after a night of not sleeping because I absent-mindedly drank a coffee, the intense feeling of grief hit me. As painful and shocking as this experience was, it needed to happen the way it did. I was very deluded about what a relationship with her could be like. I wouldn't have had it go any other way. I needed to learn the value of accepting impermanence, that love is chemical and therefore not consistent, and that I mustn't get so emotionally invested when clearly I could see the signs. I wanted to be happy so much so that I was willing to be ignorant to what I already knew to be true. I also could not expect emotional consistency and support from her because I myself could not have been emotionally consistent or supportive.

In the end, I got what I wanted out of the psychedelic experience. I definitely developed philosophically and used the experience to understand myself and my own spirituality. I would like to do mushrooms again but I think I need to wait awhile. My values and my notions of reality were profoundly altered. I enjoyed the experience of delving into my psyche and having conversations with my subconscious. It was very necessary for me as a being to experience an expansion of consciousness. I will attempt to integrate what I learned into my normal stream of consciousness, but I don't imagine that will come easily.

EXPERIENCE WITH THE DIVINE MOTHER

Ayahuasca

Being born in a spiritual land, ever since I was a child I had always wanted to see the other side, to receive powerful communications from another realm, and to return to this existence as a strong spiritual warrior. I got the idea to experience Ayahuasca after watching several documentaries about it, reading blogs, consistently hearing tales of life-changing experiences and witnessing divine encounters of this healing plant by indigenous tribes and shamans.

I had heard that setting an intention for the medicine would give me the best effects, so my intention with the Ayahuasca ceremony was to "heal" any ancestral karmic debts and patterns lingering. I came to the sacred medicine with respect, reverence, and good intentions, not to mention my passion for experiencing different realms of consciousness. Experimenting on our own psyche leads to a broader understanding of the subjective world we inhabit. This has been my main drive to experiment with consciousness on a personal level. It has led me to meditation, yoga, Qigong, fasting, lucid dreaming and the most important of all, mindfulness in my physical daily life. Overall, I realized this physical existence is the reality I have to face, since finding my life in alternative states of consciousness can be just another easy escape to keep me from facing my true self.

I was asked by a good friend to join on her this journey and gladly joined, as I was afraid to do it on my own. The ceremony was a two-day gathering and most of our group would turn out to be Ayahuasca virgins. When we arrived at the venue, I met the Shaman. His face was powerful, radiant, warm, and wise, but most of all loving and kind. We had our gear with us and the set up was ready. Our Shaman explained the process to us and asked that we set an intention for our ceremony. Mine was to find deeper direction of my life purpose and calling.

The setting was peaceful and Zen. An altar was created, candles were lit, and the area was smudged and cleansed. There was a meditation and prayer. When our Shaman handed the cup to me, my arms started twitching, my mind was racing, and my ears were ringing.

Most people who take part in several Ayahuasca ceremonies will experience at least one Ayahuasca purge. You could say an Ayahuasca purge is a bit like a car service for a human being. An Ayahuasca purge usually involves a lot of vomiting (and sometimes a lot of shitting) but you're not just ejecting physical stuff. The purge clears you of all the toxic energy and emotions that have clogged up your system, usually being carried by you unknowingly. I know that sounds a little bit gross, and it's true that purging is never fun or pleasant; however, it's ALWAYS extremely worth it. Often after purging you feel like you've been given a brand new body and you feel a profound sense of well-being that often lasts for many days, weeks, or even months afterwards. Just like your car feels like new after a good service, your whole being can often feel new after a good

Ayahuasca purge.

Forty minutes after ingesting the tea, the uptake of DMT to my brain started altering my perception of reality. I had visions where the Ayahuasca mother spirit spoke to me, giving me knowledge about my hidden unconscious psyche. The Divine Mother Ayah showed me a visualization of my past. I was shown images of my childhood and different family members distant and close, some of whom I had never even met in person, followed by intense, bright visualizations. I was shown beautiful geometric patterns that were swirling, changing, intertwining, and flowing.

After a while I got a hint of the essence of awareness. The best description would be that while I looked around, everything looked back. I thought I understood it then, but I quickly lost it. I had some personal "openings." I was shown situations where I realized I had to come to an agreement with myself to be more forgiving and loving, to show more empathy, and not judge myself whatsoever. My sense of time was completely gone and it felt like I'd just had a glimpse of a dream world that is interconnected to our normal world.

During the first night's ceremony, I gained the most insight towards the end of the experience. As several people were going for a second dose, those brave enough (including myself) went for a third double dose to experience more. After taking my third dose, I was shown that humanity needs to remember that this physical lifetime is an experience of love, joy, forgiveness, compassion, and acceptance, which are our true essence. Remembering all that allows us to strip away our Ego and let go of the layers of junk, excessive materialism, and greed that people pursue!

I had a vision of the traditional Shipibo textile design from Peru: geometric patterns so often found embroidered on clothes and tapestries. The designs got smaller, shrinking down to the point that they were barely visible. It was then that I realized that somehow this pattern constitutes the underlying fabric of the material Universe as we know it. Many myths speak of a web of matter that's spun together by some deity or another, which binds everything, and out of which the physical world was created. The Alchemists might call this the Prima Materia. Plato speaks of geometric archetypes (the Platonic solids) that constitute the root of everything we witness on a day-to-day basis, and philosophers throughout the ages have all maintained that numbers, shapes, and symmetry are the only things that truly matter, since they function as a kind of divine language, speaking to us of the things of God – sacred geometry. All of these thoughts flew through my mind as I watched the shimmering, Shipibo design slowly fade out of view.

Suddenly, I found myself standing next to some kind of large transparent tube, through which a variety of long, green serpents were rapidly moving. The tube emptied out into what felt like outer space. I vaguely remember seeing clusters of yellow and white galaxies, spiraling out and glowing with incredible intensity. As I watched, the threads combined and gradually merged with one another into the classic double helix form. Suddenly they were no longer threads, but vast amounts of coiled strands of DNA. I was told to keep watching, and suddenly the

DNA blossomed and expanded into a shape that I can't even describe, but was vastly more complex than our own genetic material. I felt as though the double helix was multiplied by six or seven, and the individual coils were beautifully connected, radiating outward, mimicking the galactic spirals in the distance. It was as though I was being shown the biological makeup of a being far more advanced than me.

Still surrounded by the breathtaking expanses of the Universe, some gigantic hand pulled a canopy over me and created a brand new environment. It was entirely crystalline, and composed of enormous trees that towered above my head with some kind of unidentifiable fruit hanging down, just out of reach. The whole scene glittered like a diamond. The trees were in ordered rows and felt like they were constructed out of enormous precious stones that refracted light from an unseen source. Throughout most creation myths worldwide, you'll find an island, the place where everything initially came into being. The Japanese refer to the jewel trees of paradise, and it's found in The Epic of Gilgamesh described as The Garden of the Sun, the Bible, Indian religious epics, and on, and on. In the past, on numerous occasions, I've referred to Ayahuasca as "tangible mythology." Experiences like this one are why.

This was where I lost the chronology of my experience. At some point, I was laying on my back, staring up at the ceiling and listening to the Shaman's music. My hands occasionally seemed to take on a life of their own during the ceremony. They started moving, dancing almost, looking serpentine, and kind of slithering this way and that. I stared at my right hand, painfully aware that I was the embodiment of the stereotypical "tripper" at this point, and it started to disintegrate. I saw pieces of it just kind of fly away. It reminded me of how fleeting the physical truly is, and how foolish and short-sighted I can be when I'm caught up in it.

As my hand continued to dance there in front of me, it began to beckon to a corner of the ceiling. My eyes were open throughout all of this. Suddenly, from that corner, a hole seemed to open up and light came through and connected with my head. Following the light, a golden-yellow bridge extended out and appeared to connect with the area immediately above my eyes. It felt like the light was carrying information of some kind and that it was inserted directly into my brain or my consciousness. There were vague shadows of figures at the far end of the bridge that I could barely make out. They seemed to be motioning to me. I was reminded of the Bifrost rainbow bridge from Norse mythology, connecting the world of the gods to the world of men. When whatever was happening was accomplished, the bridge retracted, the light receded, and the portal closed. I don't know what information was deposited in my head, but I was left with a strong suspicion that an enormous serpent had given birth to the world.

Then, I was placed in the center of a giant circle, which itself was situated in some kind of nebulous, red-tinted version of outer space. I focused on the point of the circle directly ahead of me, and suddenly my eyes divided, each moving around the side of my head in opposite directions, tracing the limits of the circle surrounding me. This was an odd physical sensation. As my eyes met in the back of my head, they joined together and came up and over, following the medial longitudinal fissure of the brain that divides it into two hemispheres. They followed that path until coming to rest just between my eyebrows, where I felt a very interesting, activating sensation of my "third eye." The lesson here was that in some sense the observer creates duality. Without our perception it wouldn't exist. And yet that begs the question: why are we made to perceive in a dualistic fashion? It might be a chicken-and-egg situation. What I feel comfortable saying is that there is a relationship between the circle and duality. It's a general statement, I know. I have yet to figure this particular vision out completely. It may just be something felt that's beyond communication.

The next day I was in a very good mood. I was really looking forward to what the plant spirit would reveal to me next. We started the second ceremony at nightfall. I stood up and walked to the Shamans to get my next dose of Ayahuasca tea. It was thick, brownish, and tasted a little sweet and sour, but less bitter than the first night. It reminded me most of the taste of licorice. I went back to my mat and tried to meditate and observe the other participants when they went to get their medicine. Waiting, exciting, fearing, fantasizing... it tasted earthy, wooden, and bitter. It was thick going down, and left a layer of mucous-like slime on my tongue and down my throat. Our Shaman burnt his Palo Santo while music played in the background.

Time stopped being relevant as I lay there. Scenes from my life flashed before my eyes. Things I hadn't thought about in years took over my thoughts. My ancestors, my mother, father, sister, brothers, uncles, aunts, cousins, friends from my childhood, and colleagues from university all flashed before my eyes. They were all incredibly sad. After about twenty-five minutes it hit, much earlier than any of the other participants and earlier than it had for me the day before. The visualizations were overwhelming, my stomach was screaming, and my body erupted in cold sweat. I felt feverish and my thought was, "Oh what have I done now?" Then the crying began. I was crying with such force that the best description would be a nuclear blast that ripped apart the fabric of everything that I ever thought was real. Intense visualizations bombarded me from every direction with such speed; I couldn't make sense of anything. Emotions erupted like a volcano. I could only gasp for air.

Thoughts were non-existent. My awareness was no longer connected to my body, the room, or this dimension. Was it even mine to begin with? I was consumed by fear and loneliness. I can only describe this experience as pure hell, and even that seems a big understatement. My first thought after what seemed an eternity was how to get out of there or to get there out of me. Ayahuasca does that to you. When I realized the complete horror I was in, I couldn't imagine an experience this cruel. I was telling myself I could handle it, which implied I wasn't convinced. "I am strong enough to stay calm and to just observe without identifying with the pure evil I am experiencing." Oh boy was "I," the Ego, wrong. It felt as if something was playing, or even toying, with me; a puppet for its sick pleasure. It took me a while to find out I was not as strong as I had believed myself to be. I was scared, lonely, and lost.

Rebirth was a shock. Slowly I started making sense of what I was experiencing. I took a drug, and as with any experience I figured, "this too shall pass." But I couldn't shed the doubt: what if the experience didn't pass? I still had no clue where my awareness was or how to get out, but I was relieved by some moments of clarity where I had thoughts that contained some meaning. Total acceptance is to give up the infinite urge to control. So I did. Then for the first time, I opened my eyes and saw the ceremony room. I desperately needed help to find my way back to common ground. The whole time I had my back turned from the whole group and was hanging over my blanket. I turned around only to find out the Shaman had been singing a personal song for me since the crying started. This strong, silent guy in daylight seemed so powerful and huge in the dark. I finally gave in and asked him for help. The biggest lesson I learned that night is that I can't do everything by myself and one is only just as powerful as the support of the people behind them. I feel like I had to experience this to understand that it doesn't matter how strong you believe yourself to be. Opening your heart and asking for help is, in many situations, the best thing you can do. The only thing that holds you back is your own Ego, fear, and shame.

I saw and felt the pain of humanity. I saw the pains of mothers, and I saw the suffering of losing loved ones to war. Time remained irrelevant. My mind was so clouded by dark clouds of anger, fear, regret, shame, and guilt. Scenes from my soothing words, I felt a glimpse of love breaking through the madness. A small opening up. The relaxing of a grip. I was transported back to my childhood and felt the love of my mother, and then this turned to the love of the Shaman and the people around me. Then to just love, where human beings are an instrument to express it if they can open themselves up for it, trust it, have faith in it, and love themselves for it. Love, joy, and forgiveness are the glue that makes us stick together.

I felt a deep-rooted empathy for the natural world. I saw the interconnectedness of the world, I saw the air we breathe and the food we eat becoming us. A child knows these facts, but when the magic is banned from our perception when we grow up and become "individual persons," we tend to forget. We tend to forget that the trees are our extended lungs and the rivers our extended veins. This is not the right time to delve into the depths of consciousness, but as never before I felt connected to the Earth that is our birthplace. There was something of me in all and something of all in me. I felt the love for which nature sacrifices itself, offering its own life for our benefit. And I felt the sadness and the disappointment of the ongoing abuse of natural resources, where we don't see the spirit in the forests and the mountains but see them as wood and ore waiting to be mined and plundered for profit.

Then, in the darkness of my inner vision, colors in long wispy lines, like gentle rainbow vapors, began to appear. The lines moved in and out of themselves and appeared to be lined with gear teeth moving in impossible ways. I know now that these were the classic visions of DNA reported by other drinkers. The colors became gradually brighter and the visions became more intense and beautiful as I realized this was going to be far more than just some residual effect. The images became ever more beautiful and intense, surpassing any of the comparatively graceless visuals of other drugs, and I realized my body was slipping into sensations of ecstasy more sublime than anything I had ever experienced. As the experience grew ever more powerful, the beauty of it became absolutely overpowering. I wanted more, and became ever more immersed in indescribable gratitude and utter joy such as I had never even hoped to know.

Tears began falling silently, and I remembered again asking to be relieved of my long karmic debts and to receive help to be a better person. The euphoria was so complete, it was as if I had been granted heaven itself, washing away the long years of darkness I had groped through. I was astonished that the brain was capable of experiencing such wondrous and complex imagery and of knowing such utter joy. In the midst of this, my ability to think was amazingly intact. As the intensity became ever more overwhelming, I realized I was losing awareness of my body altogether into a more shamanic dimension. I mentally called for more and more, and the ecstasy and gratitude that followed seemed infinite.

Then the lessons came. They came from a hidden presence of relentless tenderness I had experienced before, only now the presence had a new power and depth. I saw what could be called entities of immense beauty, but knew not to mistake images of things for the reality of something existing outside my drugged brain. Telepathically they said that I had spent most of my life running away from my own pain, manipulating and defending, sleeping, doing anything but experiencing the natural pain of being a human being. The gratitude I was feeling was indescribable. It filled my entire being, as the ecstasy also became absolute suffering at the same time, and I was infinitely grateful for both. The light became sacredness, pain, ecstasy, and beauty as one. I found myself weeping, feeling all these emotions at once, as if I had been emotionally dead for years and was now suddenly able to feel again. Great, warm, wide rivers of tears flowed in gratitude, release, and realization that I had been so cold and angry inside for so long and was now alive and able to feel again. The weight of how I had acted with my family during the years of depression flooded over me and I sobbed heavily for not being grateful and cherishing all those years. I was hallucinating, but that was opening my emotional centers. I realized this was the idea behind doing Ayahuasca.

I tried to lie quietly through the rest of the experience. We lay together quietly for the next five hours while the rest of the experience ran its course, gradually tapering off, giving ecstasy, pain, and insight. Finally, when I was relatively down, we slept. The experience lasted a bit over nine hours and felt like an eternity. The next day, I was grateful for my life and for my family. I enjoyed parts of my life I had previously considered a burden. Working became easier and enjoying simple pleasures seemed natural, instead of almost impossible. The experience of not being worried and being emotionally normal again was beyond anything I hoped for.

My encounters with La Madre relativized my Ego – that is, take it off center stage, diminish its tyrannical aspects, and have a greater sense of my wider psyche. What a great relief! I believe that one of the greatest gifts from Ayahuasca is a deeper appreciation of life. The connection that Ayahuasca often helps you feel makes you far more deeply appreciative of nature, life, and the Universe, and how it's all interconnected. I finished each of my Ayahuasca ceremonies with an overwhelming feeling of gratitude for my life and for all the people who are in my life.

The question of "Who Am I?" has probably been asked by every spiritual seeker who has ever walked the Earth. You can spend an entire lifetime trying to answer that question and still feel like you're not getting any answers. I can't say that Ayahuasca will answer the question for you, but it will almost certainly reveal many things about you that you may not have been consciously aware of. It helps to strip away all the many layers of bullshit, materialism, and Ego that often cloud our judgment and prevent us from knowing our true selves.

We are all products of our social conditioning. As we grow up, our friends, family, religion and society have a huge influence on the type of people we become, and in many ways our social conditioning is what molds our perception of reality. Overcoming social conditioning is a huge challenge for many people who often aren't even aware it's a problem. Ayahuasca allowed me to see how I've been conditioned; particularly the aspects of my conditioning that are harmful to my spiritual growth. Only through knowledge and awareness can we then start to break the conditioning that is holding us back from being all we can truly be. I have broken free from the shackles of religion and social conformity.

I've had some time to process the Ayahuasca ceremonies now. I've noticed some serious benefits since my ceremony. First, I am incredibly more present. My mind is sharper and more focused on the moment. Before, I would normally zone out every few minutes, then catch myself and try to bring myself back to the present. Since I arrived back, my mind has wandered a lot less. I have been paying a lot more attention to other people, and the scenery and sounds that surround me. Also, I felt so much fear, anger, guilt, and shame when I was on Ayahuasca. So much so that I am not scared of anything right now. I have been checking in with my emotions more frequently. About every twenty minutes I stop, ask myself, "What am I feeling right now?" and then focus on the inside of my chest where I feel my emotions. I have also been noticing other people's emotions much more since the ceremonies. My own emotions have also been much stronger and more vibrant. I feel that emotional intelligence is one of the most amazing aspects of being human and it is a strength everyone should work hard to develop. I've been concentrating on creating love in all of my interactions with others and being a helpful friend to everyone.

One of the big reasons I wanted to do Ayahuasca was because I wasn't happy with my sex life. Sex and sexuality have always been a big topic for me. I've long felt that I used sex improperly. It was more of a medication to avoid a feeling rather than a celebration of a beautiful relationship. Since coming back I have looked at men, my body, and sex differently. I am treasuring the sacred union of sex as a spiritual connection rather than just looking at sex as a physical act.

After seeing how people are suffering around the world during my experience, simple things like food, running water, and electricity make me feel so grateful. I am so incredibly blessed that I was born the way that I was and for all the people in my life. Seriously, I love the people in my life so much. My Ayahuasca ceremonies were some of the scariest, most powerful and revealing experiences of my life. I struggled quite a bit with many demons I had been ignoring or suppressing. I dealt with a lot of them. Now, my job is to make sure this doesn't go to waste. To continue to eat healthy, journal every day, meditate, love others, and continue to be of service as much as possible.

One of the biggest realizations I had is that drugs do not hold the answer. There is no escape! They cannot give me what I seek. They can help, that's for sure, but they will not make me consistently feel peace, love, and understanding. They're only messengers. It's up to me to do the work. The only way I have discovered to do that is to serve others and not worry about myself. It's really hard to be nervous when my mind is on service.

Since all this I've been living lighter and happier. The world has become dreamlike with endless possibilities. The philosophical implications of experiencing an awareness not fixated on these forms are mind breaking and I am slowly opening up to what the sages, shamans, and mystics of all ages have been saying since the dawn of language. Will I do it again? Yes. If you're looking for a sacred healing experience, I highly recommend Ayahuasca.

A COLORFUL BUDDA

Psilocybin

One summer day I consumed a Psilocybin chocolate equivalent to about 3.5 grams of dried mushrooms. About twenty minutes after consumption I began to feel a gentle intoxication come on in the form of an enhanced sense of color. I walked outside to feel the sun and surrounding woods, enjoyed my slightly altered state of perception, and had a feeling that this experience was going to be a bit stronger than I had anticipated. As I came up, my body began to feel as if it had an energetic lightness to it. I felt as if I had an unlimited amount of energy and my limbs felt slightly tingly all over.

I was enjoying the rapid come up and noticed an old trampoline nestled back at the edge of the yard where the woods began and felt called to jump and play around on it. After playfully jumping around and enjoying my dreamlike perception, I lied down to relax and look up at the trees and sky. The trees pulsated, causing me to laugh and smile, and I closed my eyes to relax and enjoy the sun's warmth once again. After a few moments, the sunlight's redness behind my eyelids began to dance and morph into different geometrical shapes and images. Watching more intently, faint lines began to dance and form into intricate kaleidoscopes of all sorts of color and forms. After a few minutes of watching the incredible patterns within my head, I became totally immersed, completely forgetting I was on mushrooms or lying on the trampoline and only aware of the beautiful colorful geometric patterns swirling behind my eyes.

Suddenly, the swirling patterns came to the form of a massive colorful finger pointing directly at me. The tip of the finger took up the entirety of my vision, and then, in incredible detail, the finger retracted and revealed itself to belong to what appeared to be a massive Buddha sitting cross-legged in front of me. Now, I was raised Christian and didn't consider myself religious at the time, but the feeling I had while observing this peaceful being was that this was the infinite source of the Universe, what most call God. Still shocked, I exclaimed, "It's you! I can't believe it's you right in front of me! You are God!" I was hoping for it to speak or acknowledge what I was exclaiming, but the Buddha only offered a gentle and loving smile back. At this time I noticed what appeared to be twenty to forty other colorful fractal-like figures emanating from behind the Buddha to form a flying V formation with the Buddha at the front. Still in awe, I suddenly received a very clear and strong intuitive thought that, "Everything is One" and that "Everything around me was profoundly connected in ways that I didn't yet comprehend." This epiphany felt so pure and truthful that I felt it in my very core, and a wave of peacefulness and love washed over me.

Shortly after, my eyes fluttered open to reveal the trees and sky. I was shocked at first, then remembering that I was lying down on a trampoline; I was equally startled, realizing what I had just experienced. It took a few moments to comprehend what had just happened and then a few more moments to let everything sort of sink in. I jumped up on the trampoline, excited to share this experience with a friend of mine, but quickly remembered that I was still under the influence of mushrooms. Realizing that I had just gone through a powerful drug-induced experience, I developed a newfound respect and appreciation for mushrooms and their potential influence. Shortly after this reflective moment, I popped up on the trampoline and quickly jumped off, hurrying over to my friend who was also enjoying the effects of the psychedelic chocolates.

I was still feeling profoundly peaceful and humbled from what I had just experienced but was also very excited in sharing the visuals and epiphany I'd just had, as we were both relatively inexperienced with psychoactive drugs. I found my friend nearby enjoying the sun and visuals she was having. I began to passionately explain the series of events that had just taken place, when unbeknownst to me a spider began to descend from one of the tree branches directly above. My friend took quickly took notice and warned me, exclaiming, "Look out for that spider!" At that point in my life I had borderline arachnophobia and would have normally jumped out of the way in fear of the spider. However, I was still retaining a great deal of peace and a sense of Oneness from my experience. I gently watched the creature lower down onto my shoulder and acknowledged its existence. It meant me no harm and I had no reason to be afraid, as it was simply being a spider and I just happened to be underneath it while it decided to lower down. I felt a great peace and connectedness with this small arachnid in realizing it was just another being of life that was simply trying to live. I held the sense that this was another being in a different form rather than a terrifying and hairy spider with many legs, fangs, eyes and whatnot. We were two beings of life that cohabited the same sea of creation, separate yet one and the same in an essence. I possessed no fear in my consciousness while I slowly bent down and picked up a stick to carefully lift the spider off of my shirt and safely place it in the grass, away from where we might step on it. My friend's jaw dropped knowing how afraid I normally was of spiders and she eagerly awaited my story and epiphany that had caused such a change of character within me.

This experience was profound to me in that it expanded my consciousness to possibilities that I had never considered, giving me a newfound respect for altered states of consciousness and how they can positively affect your waking life. I also lost a large part of my fear of spiders that day and today my fear of spiders and other "creepy crawlies" no longer exists. Ever since then, I have retained a portion of that sense of Oneness, and the experience has guided me down a more spiritual path in search of what life is really all about and what is truly possible.

THE AWAKENING

Psilocybin

Most human beings alive today are being controlled but have no idea! We live in a simulation, because the matrix is reality. The asleep believe in the system, for they are being told numerous lies, and it brainwashes them. The modern American nation is a movie. The corporation that is the United States of America constantly invades other countries; they are responsible for countless deaths, and hide subliminal messages inside of American movies. This all happens right in front of the population's face, yet the chances of them finding out are close to none. They believe too much in the system for them to believe in some "conspiracies."

Magic mushrooms have changed my life. There is a spiritual awakening happening right now as we speak. Before my experiences, I was highly Atheist and only believed in science and factual data, but soon realized science can be a part of spirituality. I have kept growing stronger spiritually, allowing myself to have fascinating experiences. One of the most intense experiences happened one night when I took 4.4 grams of Amazonian Cubensis, a strain of Psilocybin mushrooms. I chose double-four because this constantly occurring angel number has been the inspiration towards advancing my future. The number four also occurs the day of my birth, being born on October 4th, and has been influencing my life for the greater good.

I am used to tripping, so it just started as a normal trip. I was smoking marijuana to amplify the effects of the trip. This trip was especially intense, which was weird since I have taken bigger doses. I was about to go out for the night, but that never happened. This trip was different. My consciousness felt maxed out, where only my mind was functioning correctly. My physical functions were abnormal, so I decided to meditate, which made me feel alive. I felt as if I really had a purpose on this planet and I sat on the bed loving every moment that passed.

As my eyes closed, I was able to feel the horizon line, which allowed me to control the line. This feeling, while difficult to explain, allowed me to control the environment around me and feel all of the energy. The energy around me felt alien-like and I no longer felt as though I was in the same room that I was meditating in. This part is also difficult to explain, however my meditation allowed myself to "hack" through space, where I saw different lights zooming past myself. This phenomenon occurred quickly, but it felt as if the world wasn't moving. I believe the still frame in my life allowed me to control the environment even more, since my consciousness was maximized.

I soon awoke in a computer room, feeling lightheaded and drowsy. My vision was a little blurred, as if I were just knocked out. I was able to see, just as I would normally see in the virtual world. This room was small; however, the room I saw was surrounded by glass and it seemed as if the room was soundproof. Unable to move, I awoke to a man and woman who had the facial expressions of a person who just saw a murder. The shock on their faces was accompanied by the words, "Oh my god, he is awake!" My reaction was the same as when I was meditating; I was not fearful of what was occurring, yet the computer scientists I saw were frightened. I was unable to look down to see if I had a body or legs, however, I felt as if my body was half machine. I could only feel my consciousness growing, and I could only see. The rest of my functionality was still unknown to me. I felt as if my body was open and they were operating on me. I was able to see a flashing red light emanating from where my body would have been. The light was synchronizing with a loud factory alarm, almost as if something horrific just happened. I felt the presence of more individuals surrounding us, but I couldn't see them. The two individuals in front of me were on computers, which to me seemed like the main CPU of the simulated world we live in. I theorize this might be the same for all humans on Earth. These people were in distress since they saw I awoke, and were typing a hundred miles an hour, using their technology to knock me out again.

The whole experience, which happened so quickly, ended with me transferring to my body in the dormitory where I was meditating. I was mind blown and happy at the same time, wondering what had just happened. I was a bit concerned because I didn't know where I went or what this world really was. I also theorize that this place we are in is something so different. I had the realizations that this different memory location that I traveled to has influenced me and that we live in some sort of super computer. Everyone's consciousness is linked to the source which gives us consciousness, also known as God, which allows us to create the world by reflecting our perception of life.

During my experience, my mind was in control and allowed me to wake up back in the room I was meditating in.

During the trip I was calm, allowing my positive mind to keep me safe. This is a common law, known as the Law of Attraction. We can create our world both mentally and physically, which is great for accomplishing anything. I am using this mental process for completing my Computer Engineering major and believe this major has influenced my thought process, ultimately leading me toward this experience. I believe that the Elite are covering up something so complex, which explains the movie-like world. The Matrix was a movie to show the citizens what the world really is, but the Elite know this only makes the masses believe it is a movie, and nothing more. We are all here for a reason and are living in a world controlled by lies, but can be saved with the power of God. When the mind of every individual is positive, the world will change for the greater good of humanity.

THE GREAT ARCHITECT OF LIFE

LSD

There is no way to tell my story without coming off utterly insane. However, I truly believe this experience was not only life-changing, but was a major awakening and change in my life and soul. I consider myself a Shaman – an explorer of spiritual and psychical realms. I've seen many things, although nothing will ever compare to this truly humbling and enlightening experience. It all started with LSD...

My two friends and I had decided that we would not only push ourselves to a higher consciousness, but test our mental and spiritual limits. One friend had similar goals in mind, as we are both very spiritual and experiment with LSD for spiritual purposes only, however, my other friend uses it strictly for recreational uses. I planned to take two hits of LSD every twenty minutes, which eventually dosed to fourteen LSD hits. The others took seven hits, as I am much more experienced. Each dose had approximately 400 micrograms, which equals to about four hits per one hit. Overall, I consumed 5,600 micrograms of LSD.

Everything was going smooth. We simply enjoyed ourselves, laughed and had a great time until I planned to meditate. First I made sure the others were safe. It all hit me unexpectedly. I was staring at my friend, who at this point turned into a midget and ran off. I was far gone, but doing well. When this happened, I burst out into laughter and felt nothing but complete joy. After a good two minutes of laughing, my laughter turned into tears. At this point I felt many things, as I was curled up into a ball on the couch. In a matter of one second on Earth, and what would feel like hours in this realm, I belonged to this being I believed to be God.

I was face-to-face with him, though he was a blinding humbling light, weakening and bringing me feelings of utter joy, sadness, fear, and even humbling bliss. I can hardly explain this feeling, other than that it was divine. At this point, I felt that I was in two places at once; in the presence of this God, and on Earth completely conscious of both of these worlds. In this, I was scolded by this being for being so misled and blind. I remember the conversation with this being and feeling that I was with him for hours, even though on Earth it happened in a split second.

After being scolded, he revealed to me many truths and falsehoods that haunted me. I could never fully describe this experience, other than that it was the most humbling experience that I had ever had. When this being explained everything, I began to see the Architect of the spiritual and psychical plane, and how this being had created EVERYTHING. I walked through this spiritual grid that had lines everywhere. There were numbers and so much math, it blew my mind. Everything made so much sense. This is what I believed to be God's Architect. It was all too organized and structured too perfectly to be a fabrication of my mind. This was not in my head. It was real.

In this moment, my friends were observing me, seeming very interested in everything. I tried so hard to describe everything to them, all while walking psychically in this grid-like world. Suddenly, a being came into my presence. He was formed like a grid, similar to a 3-D model in a video game before they place the skin on the character. This man guided me using a conscious voice and as we walked a world began to form around me. What appeared before me was similar to a library. Upon seeing this, I knew exactly where I was – the Akashic records. In this moment, an unlimited and overwhelming source of knowledge poured through my mind at an unbearable rate.

Suddenly, spiritual truths and Earthly visions ran through my head at the speed of light. At this point, I knew I was connected to an unlimited source of knowledge. On Earth, my friends surrounded me, as I kept spinning in a circle while walking through this library. I was spitting out countless amounts of information that for some reason only made sense to my spiritual friend who had experienced this himself. I felt like I knew everything. Any question asked was answered, no matter how difficult. Even now, I can recall this knowledge very easily, as I feel I am now connected to this place by soul.

I felt countless emotions and saw the most horrifying visions of pain and suffering, as well as beauty. I saw all aspects of the Earth and grew more spiritually aware the longer I dwelled in this library. After a few minutes, everything grew more rapid and intense. Everything was infinite and way too much for my human mind to handle. It started to hurt and became so overwhelming. I forced myself out in tears and the felt so many emotions within a second. Again, one second on Earth was like hours there. I can't explain...

I tried to describe so much, but there were no words to describe such divine knowledge. I saw this vast knowledge and was only revealed a fraction of it. It blew my mind how massive and infinite everything was. Countless visions and voices, running forward and backward in time. After I left the Akashic records, due to the immense intensity, I started walking through many different dimensions simultaneously, witnessing countless beings and worlds, all of which were as conscious of me as I were of them.

In this moment, I experienced this feeling of becoming one with everything, and realized that EVERYTHING is one. All lives, beings, even a simple rock. We are one. I cannot describe it. At this point, my mind was worn and blown away and I needed a break. I needed to fathom everything, because it was all too much to handle.

I know some who have had a similar experience, which ensures my faith that this was all 100% real and divine. Now, I am a changed man. I see the world with more sympathetic eyes and with a much deeper connection to everything. I now hold a connection with this being, and he guides me. I do not share all this for bragging rights. That is not my reason. I share this because I feel that I have been given a privilege of viewing this amazing experience. I want the world to know that their spirit is more real than they could ever imagine and that although there are many gods, there is ONE above all. I am also hoping that I just might find someone who can relate to all of this. I'm sorry that I can't be more vivid, but remember, I have only shared with you a small portion of my experience and described everything the best I possibly can.

Source: https://www.shroomery.org/13620/The-Great-Architect-Of-Life-5600-UG-Experience

A LIFE CHANGING EXPERIENCE

Psilocybin

My story begins a year ago when I ran across the Johns Hopkins study on Psilocybin. Having suffered for years with depressive episodes, mild PTSD, slight bipolar tendencies, and general anxiety and unhappiness, I read the study results and then read everything I could find. I joined the discussion boards, read the trip reports, and studied McKenna and Watts. I became an avid student of the mushroom. Having tried for years to find a solution to my mental strife with traditional medicines with no success, I was captivated. I had thought mushrooms were just a fun party drug that we left behind after our college party scene. However, being open-minded, and having nothing to lose, I embarked on a journey to self-enlightenment and repair of my psyche.

I grew my mushrooms, and then carefully planned the set and setting. I meditated and I prayed to the God I thought I knew and to the God I was yet to meet, to carry me through this 5-gram, in-the-dark, scary-as-hell experience that was about to commence. About thirty minutes after consuming the mushrooms, I started seeing fractals, colorful and intricate, like nothing I had ever seen in this life or could even imagine. They were insanely beautiful, and they were alive with their own spirit and knowledge. I had headphones with Pink Floyd on and the visuals began to sync with the sound, and I was lost in it. At sixty minutes I was pinned to the couch, feeling like was I was being overrun by a succession of tsunamis, each one bigger that the one before. I was moaning and sweating and curled in the fetal position. My last coherent thought was that I was going to miss my son, because surely I was about to die. And so I did.

Time lost all meaning, my body was gone, the present was gone, and I was dying. But the death was only a massive deprogramming. All the knowledge, all the habits, all the history, all the life experiences, all the bias and the cynicism, and all of the walls I had built over this lifetime were being disintegrated. I remember my soul being beaten like I was in a cosmic washing machine. My psyche was being thrashed and pounded and my understanding of myself was being ripped away. All I thought that I was, and all that I thought I understood, was but one tiny experience in an infinite number of experiences – and it almost meant nothing.

This mental beating went on for what seemed like eternity. I struggled and I resisted, and I kept being pounded against the cosmic rocks. Then there came a point where I just let go and welcomed what I now know to have been my Ego dying. Complete Ego death – the Ego that had taken my infinite conscience and held it prisoner behind bias, ignorance, experience, and fear. I came to accept that my "life" was but a way station, a single blink of one experience in an infinite universe of experiences.

As my mental walls finally came down, I was told by the Universe itself that it was okay. It is okay. All is okay. So I let out a long breath and I let go. I was nothing, and I was everything. I was creation and I was infinity, and it was orgasmic. I remember floating in space, spinning and smiling, and I clearly remember thinking that nothing has ever felt this good. This was who we are – we are bliss. And we are good, and strong. I cried for relief, and I knew for sure and deep in my bones that things have always been and would always be okay. I am okay. I was reduced to only consciousness, floating freely in the Universe. I was it and it was me, and yet I was nothing. I apologized over and over for the hubris that had defined all of my actions on this Earth.

And then it happened. I was reborn back into myself. And I was shown that birth is what it is all about – death and rebirth, over and over again. The death was a crushing of the constructs we have built during our "life," and birth was what the root and goal of our consciousness is about. I experienced my birth – and words simply cannot describe that. I was overwhelmed in ecstasy. Nothing could possibly compare to this feeling. As the mushrooms slowly let me go at 5 AM or so, everything was clear. I was calm and very happy. Life made sense, and I was at complete peace. It was like a cosmic roto-rooter had scrubbed my conscience of all the sludge that was slowly killing me, holding me back from living.

Since then, several months have passed and I divorced the wife that was a black hole in my life for reasons that would take many more pages to explain. Suffice it to say that I was given a crystal clear directive to eject this psychic vampire from my life, and so I did. Also, since then the resistance that has defined my life for as long as I can remember has lessened. When I get into a sour mood, most of the time if I stop for a minute and reflect back on my trip while staring at the sky I can get myself centered and calm again. All aspects of my life have improved and I am becoming who I thought I could be, but by no means am I done exploring.

As anyone who has experienced the magic of the mushroom knows, it's impossible to accurately recount the experience either in person or in print. The incredible knowledge you are given and things you are shown simply wither and blow away with any serious attempt at recounting them. It's an impossibly maddening experience trying to adequately convey one's mushroom trip without looking like you have lost all your marbles. The wisdom turns against itself and defies the telling. As all of us who have traveled that path in earnest understand with no doubt whatsoever that our existence in, and interconnectedness with, the Universe makes us both nothing and everything simultaneously, significant and insignificant at the same time – one just as true as the other. Yin and Yang, ones and zeroes. Some (including myself) have said that during their trips they saw God and he is us. If you remove the brashness from that statement, it rings with staggering truth.

On one hand, we are just cosmic dust with a heartbeat, but on the other hand, we are the creator as well as the created. We contain the birth and death of all history behind us and all possible futures in front of us. We are infinite, and when we are firmly in our trips we are able to finally begin to wrap our minds around that concept. The infinite and interconnected conscience of all that IS simply feels right, it makes sense, and it is pure bliss. We now know how ignorant we have been for so long with our Egos in the way, and we are utterly humbled at the incredible beauty that we have seen. We are struck down to our knees at the magnitude of the revelations we have been shown. Our experiences granted us a level of peace and understanding that sings in our heart, even though it defies all logic and rational thought.

Source: http://www.shroomery.org/13500/Life-Changing-Experience

THE VOICE INSIDE, FEED IT

Ayahuasca

I was born to a couple that initially wasn't allowed to be together. Mom being Turkish Muslim and Dad being Armenian Christian, they weren't allowed to be together due to their individual religions and their parents' beliefs and due to the genocide, but took it upon themselves to run away and be together.

Since my parents are from two separate religions, religion has never been a big deal to me, although my sister and I were baptized at a church as part of our "christening." I didn't have the faith to believe that there are all of the different religions, but only our religion was right or true. When I was about ten years old, I often asked my father about what happens after we die, and one day he told me to ask the priest at the church. The priest was confused as to why I was even thinking about these things but went on to tell me about Heaven and Hell, and that if my belief was in Jesus I wouldn't have to worry about Hell. This only made me question it even more.

One day, my friend Jon finally told me that he'd take me to his dad's meditation center. This happened to be the same day as my cousin's wedding. I had repeatedly asked him to take me there, so I had to take this opportunity. I left my cousin's wedding after the church ceremony and went home to change.

Once we made it to the center, all I could look at was the

walls, which had all of these pictures of Buddha and other beings I'd never seen before. Everyone there treated me like they'd known me all my life. Everything felt just right while being there. Everything that Jon said had me astounded. I loved what I was learning from him and the purity of the people at the center, so I haven't stopped going since.

It was my fourth time taking part in this type of ceremony. While sitting on my mat waiting for the ceremony to begin, I observed everyone else in the group while they did their individual prayers and chanting in preparation. Being one of the first three to go up and receive the Ayahuasca, goosebumps took over my whole body knowing all too well what it tasted like. The taste can't be described but it tastes like a mix of plants, roots, and dirt – pretty much what Earth would taste like. But the taste got washed away in about twenty seconds or so with the help of a grape we ate afterwards. Today, every time I hear the word "Ayahuasca" or think about it, those goosebumps come back.

After taking my Ayahuasca, I sat back down on my mat and waited for everyone else to take theirs. After everyone had taken the medicine, they sat down in the meditation pose, relaxing, clearing the mind (or trying to), and waiting for the Ayahuasca to start working. In about twenty minutes, it did just that. It all started with random images and shapes of things that didn't make much sense, like an orange cat somersaulting, as the head of the body was standing still, then a lot of orange cats somersaulting on nothing but a black space. A short while afterwards, I had the urge to take my socks off and it felt like something was flowing through my feet. Maybe it was the voice of the

Shaman that was leading the ceremony.

At one point, all these negative thoughts and emotions came rushing to me. I thought, "This is going to be a bad experience." Refusing to have a bad experience with a bunch of good people in a safe place doing a positive thing, my positive side took over and literally said, "No, that's not going to happen today. It's not what I want." Of course the negative was persistent, causing me to open my eyes repeatedly to try to get out of that bad place, but I just kept breathing out every time there was a negative thought or energy coming to me.

The Shaman took a break from all the chanting he'd been doing with his more experienced students and started to tell a story. It was perfectly timed because the story was about getting to really know people. Not just the person we allow others to see, but the person inside that person which leads them to do the negative and hurtful things. He went on to say that we all have this other person inside us, causing us to do damage without us realizing that it is the wrong thing to do, which is the mind and the Ego.

As he was speaking about this, it felt like there was a separation inside of me and I knew what he was talking about. The first thing that happened was realizing all the worrying and negative emotions that go on inside of me on a daily basis and how they don't resolve anything. It just drains energy and puts me off from what needs to be done, not allowing me to live in the present. For the first time ever, I was able to distinguish between the two ways of thinking that most of us have. It made me realize that there is no need for negativity, anger, resentment, and most of all worry. All that those things do is keep us from enjoying life as much as we can. Most of us are also missing self-love from our lives and honestly speaking, I'm probably the worst example to give about loving myself. Loving myself? No, that didn't happen for the first twenty five years of my life. Slowly but surely my feelings toward myself are changing for the better. Of course, it's so clear to see these things while in a ceremony. It's all the times that we are not in ceremony that we need to pay attention to them. This separation allowed me to see that love really could conquer everything, as cliché as it sounds. It is the only thing that can conquer everything. Money, cars, and materialistic things aren't love; they are just things, like a piece of paper or lint from our pockets. Why do we think a car or house can make us happy when our internal process is what we really need to alter? That right there is the mind and the Ego.

The first three times doing the Ayahuasca ceremony, people in the ceremony would laugh while chanting and I couldn't seem to figure out why. That was another thing this fourth ceremony allowed me to understand. It's like us humans are all connected; not just in this ceremony, but always. This time, purely out of understanding, when they started laughing I found myself laughing with them. It's not like there was someone telling a joke or making faces. We all had our eyes closed in meditation pose, but this time I could feel what they felt, which seemed like pure fun and love, which caused me to laugh.

At one point the Ayahuasca got stronger, causing me to lie down. It showed me what seemed like a glimpse of my future. It was me standing in my office on the phone as I do on a regular basis, but this time I was looking inside from the outside at a pile of paperwork on my desk enclosed in this office, while the whole world was outside. I quickly realized that even though everyone says "I'm just doing this for now," it doesn't work like that. If you keep going, it just keeps repeating day after month after year of the same job or profession. I realized that this was not something I wanted to waste my life doing.

Another thought that came to me was the center in which the ceremony was taking place. I regularly go to the center about two to four times a week for meditation. It just felt like this was something that I could finally say I was doing right without any doubts. The center was shown to me as love, friendship, and the right path to take if I wanted to lead a positive and loving life.

Soon after, I smelled tobacco and wanted to smoke some myself. I tried opening my eyes but it wasn't so easy this time. Like I (or my spirit) was in space, speeding down towards Earth to this minuscule red dot which was my physical self. Realizing that I was in a physical body, I felt my body, hands, and feet on the floor lying down. I slowly gained movement, and then opened up my eyes. The time it took, though it may sounds like a long process, was about two to three seconds total to be able to open my eyes. I felt how small and really unimportant we are to the galaxies and universes. We are SO small compared to anything else.

The Shaman explained that just because we have a thought inside our heads, it does not mean that it is true. It is just the Ego making things up for us to believe and act upon thinking that we are right, when it's just a simple thought that we feed and make stronger. Sometimes we don't even have an explanation as to where these beliefs come from. He also said that if you can see it, it is not you, meaning that perspective, since the mind is so powerful, can show us things that we may want to see. It is our choice to dismiss an idea or thought or to feed it and let it grow. If it really was us and not the Ego or mind, we wouldn't be able to clearly see it. Most likely we will feel it, but won't see a physical image of it. In a world that judges each other by images of media, food, culture, materials, physical condition, and attributes it's very hard for us to overlook these things on a daily basis.

We all have that little voice inside of us that we usually ignore because our eyes and mind see what we think we have to have. If we just listen to this little voice inside us, even though it could be hard to hear at times, it will eventually take over and kill or dismiss the Ego, making it much easier to guide us through life.

These are all things that I've experienced and I hope that it sheds some light on the positivity that Ayahuasca can bring. Everyone at one point in their lifetime should try to have a proper Ayahuasca ceremony or if possible have two of them, since the first time you will likely just be cleansing.

HEAVENLY GOLD

Psilocybin

The tripping became more intense, to a point where I started losing control of my body. My fingers and toes were constantly twitching through my whole trip, and my left eye was completely non-operational. As I lay on the floor I could hear my friend talking, but I could not tell where the voice was coming from. In fact my senses became more and more mixed up, to the point where everything was merging into the same thing.

With my eyes closed, my surroundings transformed into the start of my voyage. I felt as if I was submerged in water – only it wasn't water, it was the very essence of space-time. It was everything, it was God. There was every emotion, every color, every moment of time and space all together and part of the same thing. I can briefly remember thinking how lucky I was to have found this state of Nirvana – and thinking of the millions of people on this planet who strive to find God through religion, but have not and never will experience such a profound feeling.

As I voyaged further, I came to a land of paradise. All matter was made of a bright light, a kind of shining gold. It was everything, infinity – this was the "pinnacle" of everything. Despite the intensity of this trip I felt as if my ego-less conscious mind was completely active. I could think rationally and question to myself what was happening. My mind was trying to find a word for the place that I was in. I thought through many words before I found the right one – an "alternative civilization," "the future," or "a fictional story"? No – all of these didn't quite fit. What was I experiencing? Heaven? Yes, heaven! The word described it perfectly. The moment I thought the word I knew, that was the place I was in. I came to find characters that existed in this heaven. They were kind of aristocratic and symbolized complete order and perfection – rulers of the land worshipped and uniformly respected by everything that resided in it.

Although there was one focal person who I later labeled "God," there were other characters, particularly a woman who was dressed very classy and was the epiphany of seduction – she was my feelings of lust! Further along the trip I came to the realization that these characters, gods, and rulers of everything were actually symbols of my personality. The seduction was most insightful for me, because it was lust – something I had been experiencing and talking to my friends about that previous night. It became apparent to me that these characters who existed in complete order and peace were actually not foreign gods. They were part of me and the heaven that I was in was MY heaven. It was ME.

What made this different from other trips was that I was far more aware of what was going on, and I was in control. I was able to ask these gods what I was to do when I left the trip. I explained that I was scared of not being able to deal with what I had seen. A comforting voice replied that I should not be scared, for it was nothing to be worried about since all I had seen was my own self; I had touched my true essence and had been able to read my soul for the first time ever.

I asked how I could be happy in my life knowing that it would always be dull compared to the heavenly state that I was in. In reply, I was shown that reality is more important than anything else whilst we are alive, and I was told to always do the best I could to achieve my potential. I was told that this trip would help me bring my life together and have better control of what I've done and who I was.

I was conflicted about the main character (me), because when I looked closely, a warm and loving family was under me. I had a loving wife, and children I was proud of. I knew I loved my wife completely, but I was still really attracted to lust. I can remember it taking me some time before I could resolve this conflict of being married to someone I loved yet seeing this "lust" and being attracted to it. In reality, I am not married, nor do I have children, yet I am with a girlfriend I love completely. I do have a problem of lusting after other people, but I have never been unfaithful. After much thought in my trip, I realized that the love for my family was greater than lust, yet lust was clearly going to be a problem for me since this character was a symbol of "me." With this conflict resolved, I felt myself leaving my heaven.

I was still unsure as to how I could deal with trying to explain what had happened. I was scared it would have a negative effect on me long-term. Once again, I was reassured and told never to forget the meaning behind it all and that one day I would return to it when I was in need of reminding what I am all about.

Source: http://www.shroomery.org/3924/Heavenly-Gold

RETURN TO WONDERLAND

LSD

As I sat on the mat laid out in the middle of the woods, I broke the tab in half. This was going to be my first LSD trip. Placing the tab under my tongue, my two friends and I sat patiently in wait of what was to come, with no idea that I'd be reentering my first DMT experience once again. The time began to move, and before I knew it I was looking up at the trees, relating myself to nature, as the shadows of trees plastered against the night's sky looking more and more like a network of nerves. I began to see what was so amazing about this drug.

As the night progressed, I decided to take another full tab. I watched the world around me and soon everything began to make more sense; colors became more vivid and shadows made patterns, as man and nature became one. We picked up and decided to move down to the lake we had camped near. On the walk, everything was dark and we became turned around quite easily, so we shifted our path and found our way.

On a lone bench sitting on the edge of a cliff, the three of us looked across the lake in amazement. We decided to roll a blunt and as we sat huddled amongst one another, with a single headlamp aiming at the hands of the person rolling, we watched every move that was made within the narrow gaze of the light. As I sat watching, I began to feel my consciousness leave my body. I began to rise above us. From a bird's eye view, I watched the three of us around this one headlamp. As seconds went by, I continued to soar higher and higher above what eventually became nothing more than a speck of light. The distance between my consciousness and my body made me feel like I was looking at a lone star in the dark. Suddenly I crashed back down to my body. The feeling was incredible, making me realize that my body is nothing more than a vessel with which I wander upon this Earth. My consciousness uses it for transformation and growth, and I realized that we are all infinite beings.

When the blunt was finished, we laid on a blanket holding one another in the cold December weather, doing nothing more than looking at the stars. We saw patterns and perfect alignments in the sky, and with the stars holding our gaze, we just spoke of the things we saw. The stars appeared to be gateways. Couples of stars aligned so perfectly in pairs and triplets. They seemed to be doors, from one evolution of mind to the next, and I began to wonder where I was in this cosmic pattern of evolution.

I closed my eyes. The colors! My god, the colors, the shapes, and more importantly, the eye! The same eye I saw during my first DMT experience. The eye looked at me again in confusion, almost as to wonder how I arrived, but welcoming me regardless. The stark white eye with a piercing blue iris looked back at me amongst a pallet of geometric shapes and vibrant colors. Accepting of my presence, it showed me more. A flower appeared, beginning to blossom. Is this the chrysanthemum everyone had spoken of? It blossomed so bright, so colorful, and so magnificent! I was mesmerized by its beauty. It opened up and expanded into the most beautiful flower I've ever been privileged to witness. It was amazing.

I opened my eyes to return to the lake. We looked out among the lake, seeing reflections of stars and trees. The trees appeared to be branching out towards the atmosphere, each one seeming like a nerve that branches toward our skin. I looked across the water and saw a network of trees close to one another and their reflection appeared to make a perfect wave pattern, almost as if you were looking at the sound waves of a recording. We had all been sharing thoughts and wavelengths with one another the entire night, and this was just another confirmation that we were on the right path.

We made our way back to the campsite and began to work on rebuilding our fire from the smoldering remnants. The three of us sat and relaxed, gradually moving from fireside to the sleeping bags and hammock.

I sat in the hammock rocking back and forth and it began to happen again. I was out of my body, except this time I was above the fire and it was hours earlier. I was witnessing our previous experience by the fire, floating above the three of us warming by the fire, talking of nature. Then time shifted forward, still floating above the fire. Minutes fast forward, then hours. I began to realize I am in control of it. I zipped through our different experiences by the fire. When I realized I could see the past, I wondered, "Can I see the future?" I tried and fast forward more, and suddenly I was sunken back into the hammock, looking at my feet covered in the blanket, rocking back and forth.

Closing my eyes, I began to see more hallucinations. The

colors, the shapes, the eye. The eye faded and it was just colors and shapes. I tried to control it and it began to fade. Then I relaxed and it returned. I realized that I was in control of this, but the key was to relax and let it come to me. Vibrant colors and shapes, meaning so much to me, they continued for a while but my body grew tired. I lied comfortably in the hammock, rocking back and forth. Small hallucinations, nature surrounding me in its beauty. My two amazing friends were lying beside me. I was happy. I began to drift off to sleep, thankful for all this wonderful experience had shown me.

LOST BODY

Psilocybin

I thought I was dead. I knew I had done it to myself, but could not for the life of me remember what I had taken, why I was dead, or how it happened. I simply knew that I had done it, and I was somehow in a galactic prison or a purgatory perhaps. The visions were plentiful, yet solemn. At this point they were mostly in black and white. I could feel my Ego being physically crushed, just like a can still full of liquid. As the pressure increased, the contents pushed "outward." Eventually this culminated in some sort of squashed feeling which I can only relate to the poor two-dimensional creatures of the sci-fi classic Flatland. I spent some time in this suffering and progressively more terrifying state.

An entity came and delivered me unbidden personal attention. I was quite relieved to see another creature, for I suspected I was one myself (although not sure). At first I was captivated by its fluid motions and methodical actions. It was moving in rhythms, doing a dance of sorts. It soon occurred to me that the "dance" it was doing involved horrifying probes of my own form, and that it was moving faster than I could comprehend while doing so. I was paralyzed. I wasn't sure if I had a body or not, but this thing was doing something to "me," which was still intact. As I concentrated more and more upon its "physical" form (which is a term I use as loosely as possible), it occurred to me that it looked somewhat familiar. Not anything I had ever seen, but close. It was a giant praying mantis, although it had mental appendages and cartoon details about it. It also looked squatter than the terrestrial version of the insect, shorter and more robust. Its many arms worked up and down my existence, probing and testing every bit. It seemed to put no effort into comforting me, yet it did through some sort of telepathy imply that it would be easier for both of us if I stopped struggling. Eventually I did, and it left.

I lost almost all physical awareness and felt my mind drifting through something resembling outer space. I saw stars and celestial bodies, but was not sure if they were as such or just molecules. The difference seemed irrelevant at that point. I knew I had a brain and a pair of lungs. I thought that was all. Imagining myself, I saw the brain connected to the lungs behind it and realized that these two organs in this array must have influenced the design of that dreaded spaceship "The Enterprise." As I charted the cosmos, I became aware that through a bit of imagining, or some similar process, I could arrange them to my own satisfaction. I found that different arrangements produced different mental states, some I had known, while others were wildly strange. Upon reflection, the impression that I had was that I was rearranging molecules that were fundamental in neuro-transmitting tasks. One arrangement of the "stars" felt similar to LSD, one to 2CB, and so forth. I was not aware of this at the time, however. I simply moved the stars according to whim, and felt pleased with the immediate physical results.

I'm not sure if it was intentional or not, but I had slipped into another "room." This was the typical round room deep psychedelics take me to. However, this time it was much larger than normal. Around the perimeter flowed the forms of creatures who looked more like cartoon drawings of dogs than anything else. They seemed Mayan in as far as they all had dragging tongues and eyes which looked only backwards. They seemed to give me a grinning, sarcastic sneer as they drifted past me.

Meanwhile, in the middle of the "sphere," I had other entities to deal with. I cannot come up with any words to describe most of them, although the frivolous doodles that cover the margins of my school lecture notes come closer than anything at approximating their forms. The only clear example I can present is one interesting specimen: I saw a Mexican man, dressed in traditional Huichole garb, kneeling and vomiting on himself. He looked up at me with a knowing glance and continued his vomiting. I wondered later if I really met him or not. I also wondered what entheogen or technique took us to the same place. It occurred to me a month or so later to wonder if he had seen a college honkey, stoned to the gills on mushrooms, floating through his own sacred space.

I finally relaxed, enjoying the inevitability of it all. Instantly, flowers looking like opium poppies surrounded me and the "machine-elves" of DMT fame came to visit. They assured me that I was safe, and a really nice guy to boot. In their high-pitched collective voice, they sang a song revealing to me not only my own nature, but that of all creatures as well. They assured me that my DNA was not only similar to their own, but part of, as well as encompassing, their own "code." They stressed the simultaneousness of this seemingly contradictory statement. I started to laugh out loud, mostly at the absurdity of it all. My laughing became uncontrollable. It should be added that at this point I was so immersed that it did not matter if my eyes were open or closed. However, this laughing was the first event, in what seemed like months, which reminded me of my personal form and body. And I laughed... I could not stop!

The laughing at one point "locked on" to a particular vocal frequency and I could not get it to budge. Indeed, I was aware that I was releasing a monotone hum. Even breathing did not seem to interfere with its clarity. I found it satisfying, and started to explore. By going with the sound, instead of trying to stop it, it grew louder and louder. Eventually it culminated in what McKenna correctly describes as a metallic buzzing sound. Very much like the sound of a cicada, but with many other elements added. I did feel as a bug making the sound, and I had an intuitive understanding of metamorphosis.

As this sound continued, I noticed it was affecting my visions. Before, the elves were rapidly and almost violently competing for my attention, each trying to show me a better toy than the last, but this incredible sound caused them to order themselves into intricate yet subtle patterns of the greatest coherency. By slightly altering the pitch of the growl, or modulating it, the patterns changed.

After some time, I could actually sculpt three-dimensional objects. I did not attempt to make a chair, or a dog, or anything like that, but rather sculptures of pure light and revolving

LOST BODY

spheres, towers of emerald surrounded by throbbing orbs of sound and love. These were the toys I presented back to the machine-elves. This ability continued for what I would (with no way of ever knowing) say was roughly a half-hour. This was the most satisfying, absurd, and enjoyable feeling I have ever had in my life. All frustrations associated with the inability to express myself were flattened. It was as if I were vomiting my soul right into the air, where it loved to dance and play.

So now I am left with a ridiculous set of goals in life. I have done this again with another person who claimed the ability, and indeed the visions were seen by both parties. Like mental sex of untold richness. The possibilities of this "language" with no danger of misinterpretation are so staggering, I can't conceive of pursuing any other future for us monkeys. To my amazement, and despite my wide sampling of the psychedelic community across the United States, this phenomenon is almost unknown. I don't know what triggers it, only that if I eat enough mushrooms it will come. Strangely, I have not been able to have much success with the vocalizations on DMT, where this supposedly manifests itself more readily.

Source: https://www.shroomery.org/4642/Lost-Body

WALK

LSD + MDMA

I tend to be the type to wait for something to feel right before delving into it. I admit this may have slowed my progress, even depriving me of experiences in some cases, but my comfort level is something I have always held dear to me. After more than a decade and dozens of psychedelic experiences, I had found the combination of LSD and MDMA, or Molly as we call it, to be the most beautiful and inviting. The LSD would open my mind, while the Molly opened my heart. This marriage never steered me wrong, so in my comfort-based mindset this would set the stage for my next journey.

After a few months of spending time together, I had become intimately involved with a friend named Lily, but we had reached a fork in the road. She was ready to walk away from our physical relationship, rightfully seeking more from someone she was openly committed to than just sex, but I wasn't ready to commit. I had planned a camping trip, but since the whole trip was really last minute just about everybody backed out. Except for Lily. She had a moment where she was also going to bail because of how she was feeling about us, but lucky for both of us she decided to come.

We had talked some time about finding the right opportunity for her first LSD experience, but less appealing opportunities came and went. Our destination was a lakefront where I had tripped before. This would be the perfect place for her to embark on her first journey.

It was a beautiful July weekend in Upstate New York. We had connected with some friends from back home and hiked to the lakefront to set up camp for the weekend, but after the first night some of the group departed, leaving me alone with Lily and our newfound friend Alex. I had no idea this day would become a pivotal moment in my life. How could I?

After spending the day exploring and relaxing on the beachfront, we headed back up to the campsite to prepare for the night. As the sun came down, Lily and I decided to take the Molly first to put our minds in a positive and joyful place. The familiar warmth of the Molly inside my chest, especially when pure, is when I know I am where I want to be. This is where I can't stop smiling, with my sense of gratitude and appreciation becoming exponentially heightened. Under the influence of MDMA, things that we normally take for granted suddenly become more beautiful not just to our eye, but to our soul. This sense of appreciation is always there, but worldly distractions tend to remove our eye from this truth.

As we approached our happy place we decided to take our first tab of LSD. Once acquainted and comfortable with the LSD feeling, we decided to take the rest of it. Lily was much braver than me, but I always loved how she respected my hesitancy and desire to do things in a way that make me feel mentally at ease. We had one sugar cube remaining, which we shared. One bite for her, one bite for me. How very romantic. Not long after, we were lying in the tent together listening to Dream

Koala, which in many ways may have led us down the path we were about to enter.

While lying on my back in the tent, I asked Lily for a hug. As she embraced me, I could feel this overwhelming sense of sadness coming from her. From our brief time getting to know one another, I knew she had overcome a difficult past. It permeated her personality in a number of ways, but as she lay on top of me I could actually feel those painful emotions emanating from her body. Physically sensing someone else's energy is something I had never experienced before. With her head buried in my chest, I could feel her crying. I knew, without knowing, what she was going through.

Lying with her, I began to hear thoughts inside my mind that I didn't recognize as my own. The voice inside my head was being answered by something foreign. With a knowing, I came to the realization that it was Lily speaking to me telepathically – or me speaking to her. Now I'm not sure, even to this day, whether we were sharing one stream of consciousness or she was just inside my head, but being a person who is logic-driven, requiring sensible evidence and explanations to be swayed in any direction, this was a complete shock to me. I had read about these sorts of things, but in all my life had never experienced it myself. And I never truly believe things until I have seen them with my own eyes.

I had known she was powerful, but I had no idea how powerful. We were both in awe. From this point forward we spent the entire night speaking without speaking. As we lied there together, still embracing, this overwhelming sense of sadness lingered so I said to her, "Give me all your pains and sorrows." Now I'm not sure what made me think or say this, but it seemed to just stream from my mind to my lips. Then again, I can't even recall if I spoke those words out loud. When I said this, I physically felt my chest open up and begin to consume this dark energy coming from Lily's body, like a transfer of energy. It felt like I was absorbing a life of pain, suffering, and loneliness into my own body. What still blows my mind to this day is that I could physically feel this happening, physically feel this energy entering my body.

Initially, I had become so focused on what was taking place that I didn't even realize what was happening. When I realized that I was actually healing her, I was able to consciously force my heart to open more, allowing more in, speaking to her telepathically saying, "Give it all to me. Don't hold onto any of it. You have to let it ALL go." As this happened, the conscious thought process occurred that I might be taking on this burden. There was a brief moment where I worried that I would be forced to experience her pain moving forward. To this day, I still don't know if it was transmuted, destroyed, or did in fact become a part of me that I now have to overcome. As this moment ended, I asked her if she wanted to go down to the lake. She regained composure and quietly nodded.

It wasn't until days later that I realized I had been wearing a black tourmaline necklace that night which she had made for me when we first met. This necklace was hanging over my heart, as it still does even as I write this. I soon came to find out that black tourmaline is known to transmute negative energy into positive energy. It's almost as if her Higher Self had instructed her to give the stone to me, knowing that I had the ability as a healer to put it to valuable use and help her along her spiritual evolution. To put her one step closer to ascension.

Even stranger, I almost immediately recalled a lucid dream that I had months earlier where I was embraced and healed by a feminine being. In this dream, I buried my head in this female's chest, upon which she had a tattoo of the Virgin Mary. She kept repeating, "I am Isis." Isis, the Egyptian goddess who searched all throughout ancient Egypt to find the body parts of Osiris in order to put his body back together and make him whole again. I felt myself melt into this female's chest, until we were one body and soul. This woman felt motherly, as if she cared deeply about what I had been going through in my life. When we embraced, I felt something open up in my chest and I consciously forced my heart wide open. I sobbed and sobbed for the purity of the love that I felt in that moment and for the absence of such love in my waking life. When I woke up, I felt lighter, as if I had experienced some sort of healing in this dream. The physical sensation of my chest opening and exchanging energy that I felt in that dream is identical to the experience that Lily and I shared. I wonder if I was being shown how to do it, so I could share this gift with others.

As we exited the tent, we woke our friend Alex who had taken a tab earlier and fallen asleep. As he gathered his things inside the tent, Lily and I went outside to wait for him. When we hugged, I could still feel that there were things she did not let go of, so we embraced, and could both feel this transfer of energy happening again. This time though I joked with Lily telepathically as it happened and I heard her chuckle out loud when I playfully said, "You have to give it all to me... I *know* you're still holding on." As we let go of each other, the reality of everything that had just happened really sunk in and we spoke about it. I guess we wanted to make sure neither of us was crazy. As Alex came out of the tent, we gathered our things for the long journey down to the lake.

It was now complete darkness, with a sky full of stars, and if there's any one activity that has stolen my heart, it is lying under a star-filled sky on LSD. We left the campsite and traveled downhill toward the lake, using only the moonlight to navigate. As we broke through thick brush, the walk down this hill felt more like we were on a journey than a simple walk. Lily and I held hands. I felt as if I was her guardian, watching over her, protecting her. In a way, I was. When we got to the base of the hill the ground leveled off. Alex had brought a wireless speaker so we could listen to music from my phone. This was perfect. Thank you, Alex.

Earlier in the night I had told them about a song by Teen Daze called "Walk." I explained to them as I have always explained this song to everyone who I've shared it with, that it sounded to me like what it would sound like walking into the afterlife. As we turned toward the lake, this song began to play. It's utterly beautiful and has always invoked in me a sense of belonging and more importantly, the emotional gratitude of finally letting go.

As we held hands and walked toward the lake, all we could

see was the silhouette of the foreground, with a large tree in the distance, and the landscape in the background, with the lake glimmering white from the reflection of moonlight. As we walked, I was suddenly pulled out of my body, observing the silhouette of Lily and me walking towards the lake in front of me. Only I was not alone. We had left our bodies together. Watching us walk together, hand in hand, I told her, "This is a rebirth." It felt as though we were walking into the afterlife together, like we were going HOME. Only it was not us. It was our souls.

While out of our bodies together I told her, "I'll always be here for you. I'll never let you fall. I love you." It felt as though we were walking down the aisle together, as we spoke to one another without speaking, making our vows. As this happened, I was not consciously aware of it or in control of what was happening, but at the same time I was completely present in it and can still remember everything about that moment. Suddenly and without warning, we both snapped back into our bodies at the exact same moment and turned towards each other and kissed. It felt like the "I do" moment. It felt like a dream.

I was completely awestruck, as I had never left my body before. I had always believed it was real, but again, I had to see it with my own eyes to truly believe it. Now back in our bodies we walked toward the edge of the lake. Within moments, Lily tripped and I caught her. I didn't mean for the whole "I'll never let you fall" thing to be so literal, but hey, it felt like something higher than us was smiling down upon us that night, almost being playful with its synchronicities. Maybe it was our higher selves looking out for us, guiding us, making sure we went down the right path. The signs were everywhere, and after that night we literally couldn't escape them.

We decided to plant ourselves at the edge of the lake and excitedly stared up at the stars as they danced above our heads. It was simply beautiful. Lily and I continued speaking telepathically, even being playful with one another and laughing out loud at what we were saying to each other. There were moments where I was having some really intense and borderline grotesque closed eye visuals and I would open my eyes in fear that she could see what I was seeing and would somehow be disgusted by it. I never understood where those types of visuals came from. When in such a perfect state of mind, completely in control of the experience, where did these dark visuals come from? It must have been something repressed deep down within my core that made its best effort to make a cameo that night. Nice try demonic morphing vaginas.

As I laid there on my back looking at the stars I could see a dome-shaped holographic grid over the Earth. I had heard of this grid before and the concept that this reality is the computer-generated manifestation of some higher form of intelligence. To bear witness to "the grid" with my own eyes, I was in complete awe.

Lily rolled over and straddled herself on top of me so we could hug. While we lay there in the grass, this intense sexual energy rose up from within me. It was the feeling that you have as you approach orgasm, but what was strange was that neither of us was physically moving. I asked, "Do you feel that?" She nodded. I focused on this sensation as it intensified and could feel our souls tangled together, as if we were two bodies with one soul. It didn't feel as though we were separate anymore and within minutes this sensation became complete ecstasy. When I closed my eyes, this orgasm became an explosion of colors and geometric patterns, almost reminiscent of fireworks. Yet we still hadn't physically moved. It was more like soul sex.

We spent hours sitting there talking about our past and the power of letting go. We made all sorts of agreements and even started naming our future children. We were excited to say the least. It's an understatement to say that this feeling is a sense of relief when you feel as though you have finally met "the one" and no longer have to search. After spending many years alone, it's easy to become hopeless and consumed by doubt, regrets, and what ifs. We could both sense each other's gratitude that night. Now, while our souls seem to have made an agreement that night, the task becomes not to allow our physical and emotional selves to fuck it up. My sense of comfort around her grew that night and I was able to completely be myself moving forward.

Writing this now, I realize that I had always felt as though it was her rebirth that night and that I was guiding her toward it, but for all I know, it was meant for both of us. Every part of me truly believes that when I die the last thing I will see is that moment, watching us walk together holding hands, and to this day all I have to do is close my eyes and I can find myself back at that lake.

Appendix

Amanita Muscaria

A. Muscaria

Famous for its distinctive white-spotted red cap, *Amanita Muscaria* is a psychedelic mushroom species found in woodlands throughout the Northern hemisphere. Also known as fly agaric, *A. Muscaria* was first documented by the Swedish botanist Carl Linnaeus in 1753. Considered a poisonous mushroom, *A. Muscaria* contains the chemicals ibotenic acid, muscimol, and muscarine, which act as deliriants. The principle psychoactive compound is muscimol, which is known to cause dissociative effects similar to lucid dreaming. However, levels of the chemicals that induce hallucinogenic versus toxic effects tend to fluctuate from one mushroom to the next.

This mushroom has been used for centuries in both religious and shamanic ceremonies in North America, Asia, and Europe. The *Rig Veda* describes an immortal and living God in the form of a drink known as Soma, which in 1968, mycologist R. Gordon Wasson purported may have contained *A. Muscaria*. Characterized in texts such as *The Sacred Mushroom and the Cross*, it is argued that this sacred mushroom is at the root of many modern religions, and is believed to have been used ritualistically for over 4,000 years. Studies have shown that these chemicals also help to turn off the part of the brain that responds to fear, effectively eliminating the recipient's fear response. It is believed that the Vikings, known as berserkers, would consume these mushrooms in order to eliminate their sense of fear during battle.

Effects can last 4-12 hours depending on potency, dosage, and delivery.

Ayahuasca
N,N-Dimethyltryptamine

Used as a religious sacrament for hundreds of years, Ayahuasca, known as the "vine of the souls," is a drink blend found in the Amazon made from the ayahuasca vine (*Banisteriopsis caapi*) and a shrub known as chacruna (*Psychotria viridis*). In some tribes, the ayahuasca vine is combined with chaliponga (*Diplopterys cabrerana*) to enhance and lengthen the experience. The brew is served in a ceremonial setting under the care of a shaman, also known as an ayahuasquero.

The DMT, which is the active psychedelic compound in the Ayahuasca brew, is found in the *P. viridis* shrub. When taken orally, the DMT is broken down by protective enzymes in the body; however, the *B. caapi* contains compounds that deactivate these enzymes, allowing the DMT to be orally active.

Users are recommended to follow strict preparations before a ceremony in order to improve their well-being and increase the effectiveness of the Ayahuasca brew, which includes, but is not limited to, no sexual activity, as well as no alcohol, fried foods, meat, or dairy. In some Ayahuasca brews, users experience fits of vomiting known as purging or "La Purga."

Scientific studies support the use of Ayahuasca in treating ailments such as addiction, Post-Traumatic Stress Disorder (PTSD), and depression.

Effects can last 2-12 hours depending on potency and dosage.

DMT
N,N-Dimethyltryptamine

First synthesized by Richard Manske in 1931, DMT is a psychedelic tryptamine compound that can be found all throughout the plant and animal kingdom, as well as within humans, endogenously produced by the brain's pineal gland. What makes DMT unique is how it is actively transported across the blood-brain barrier into the brain's tissues. However, since the body contains an enzyme known as monoamine oxidase (MAO), which breaks down the DMT, the experiences are short-lived. Another form of psychedelic DMT is *5-methoxy-N,N-dimethyltryptamine*, also referred to as "5-MeO," which is an analogue of *N,N-Dimethyltryptamine* found in natural sources such as the skin and venom of the Sonoran Desert Toad.

DMT has been used ceremonially in many different cultures throughout history, such as Ayahuasca in the Amazon where it is consumed through insufflation in the form of a "snuff" or as a brew and *Acacia Nilotica* in Ancient Egypt where it is believed that Osiris, the god of rebirth, was born from an *A. Nilotica* tree. It is theorized that the burning bush in the story of Moses' divine communication with God was an acacia bush native to that region and high in DMT content. In the early 1990's, Dr. Rick Strassman led clinical trials on DMT, where patients received dosages intravenously. During these trials, detailed in the iconic book *DMT: The Spirit Molecule*, users had very similar divine visions and encounters with beings, carrying several common themes throughout their widely varying experiences.

Effects can last 5-20 minutes depending on potency, dosage, and delivery.

Ketamine
Ketamine Hydrochloride

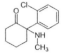

Ketamine, known for its hallucinogenic, dissociative, and sedative effects, is a fast-acting general anesthetic that has been used during surgery for both humans and animals. First synthesized in 1962 by Calvin Stevens, it was developed as an anesthetic and replacement to PCP.

In 1963, it was first patented in Belgium as an animal anesthetic and soon after, testing began on humans. That is when its hallucinogenic effects were discovered. While mainly used on animals, it has been used as a field anesthetic in military applications. Today, Ketamine is used on children and other adults during minor surgeries.

Studies have shown that Ketamine can be used therapeutically, effectively treating people suffering from major depression with an imminent risk of suicide. Furthermore, Ketamine has proven to work faster than other typical treatments, working within hours or days, while current anti-depressant medication can take weeks or months, although its effects may be short-lived.

Ketamine is typically taken intramuscularly, but can be consumed through other methods such as insufflation. During a non-fatal overdose, users experienced what is commonly referred to as a "K-hole," in which they experience detachment from reality and/or the body, as well as Near Death Experiences (NDEs).

Effects can last 5-60 minutes depending on potency, dosage, and delivery.

LSD
Lysergic acid diethylamide

In 1938, while searching for a respiratory and circulatory stimulant, Swiss chemist Albert Hofmann first synthesized LSD from ergotamine, a chemical derived from a fungus found on rye and other cereals known as ergot. It was not until 1943 that he discovered its psychedelic properties.

In Ancient Greece, a ritual known as the Eleusinian Mysteries took place every year for nearly two thousand years, where initiates would drink a hallucinogenic brew known as "the kykeon." The brew's recipe consisted of barley, often found in the fields of Eleusis infested by a fungal growth known as ergot, which also happens to be the main compound used to synthesize LSD. After the discovery of LSD, Hofmann pursued the notion that the psychedelic experience induced by the kykeon potion at Eleusis resulted from the same chemical makeup as that found in LSD.

In the late 1950's, Dr. Humphrey Osmond supplied LSD to members of Alcoholics Anonymous who had failed to quit drinking; through this, he discovered that LSD had a success rate of approximately 50% in treating alcoholism – an efficacy that had not been seen in any other type of treatment. LSD has been actively used in a therapeutic setting since the 1970's, and in more recent years it has been applied in the treatment of severe anxiety associated with terminal illness.

Effects last from 4-12 hours depending on potency and dosage.

Mescaline
3,4,5-trimethoxyphenethylamine

Found in Mexico, Central America, and South America, Mescaline occurs naturally in the Peyote (*Lophophora williamsii*) and San Pedro (*Echinopsis pachanoi*) cacti, as well as many other members of the Cactaceae family. Another well-known Mescaline source is the Peruvian Torch (*Echinopsis peruviana*).

Peyote is a small spineless cactus mainly found in Mexico and the Southwestern United States. It grows underground, where its crown, also known as a "button," can be seen from the surface. The crown, which contains the psychedelic compound Mescaline, is cut from the cactus and its buttons are dried for consumption. They may be chewed or soaked in water to create a drinkable brew.

There are about thirty species of San Pedro, mostly found in the Andes Mountains in South America, that archaeological records indicate have been used in healing ceremonies by Andean cultures for over 3,000 years.

Indigenously known as huachuma, San Pedro can be dried and ground into powder form or prepared as a brew by boiling slices of its stem. Traditionally, these ceremonies are held within the presence of a shaman, known in the Peruvian Amazon as a curandero or healer, who guides the user through their experience.

Effects can last 6-16 hours depending on the source, potency, dosage, and delivery.

MDMA
3,4-Methylenedioxymethamphetamine

Widely known as "ecstasy" for its ability to induce euphoria, MDMA is a synthetic drug that acts as both a psychedelic and a stimulant, heightening the user's sense of intimacy and emotional connection with others. With a chemical structure similar to that of Methamphetamine and Mescaline, MDMA was first discovered and patented in the early 1900's by the pharmaceutical company Merck. It was found that sassafras oil can be extracted from the sassafras tree's dried root bark through the process of steam distillation in order to obtain safrole, which is the primary precursor of MDMA.

In 1965, chemist Alexander Shulgin synthesized MDMA while performing research at Dow Chemical Company, but he was not aware of its psychoactive properties. It wasn't until 1976 that Shulgin would consume MDMA and learn about its therapeutic effects, noting that it allowed the user to see the world clearly and without inhibitions. In his pursuit to find an effective therapeutic drug, Shulgin's work influenced its widespread use in Western culture. Advocates in the fields of psychology and cognitive therapy have supported the belief that MDMA holds therapeutic benefits and facilitates more effective psychotherapy sessions by comforting the user to openly discuss deeply traumatizing experiences. Clinical trials have tested the therapeutic potential of MDMA for Post-Traumatic Stress Disorder (PTSD), as well as anxiety and depression associated with terminal illness.

Effects can last 2-6 hours depending on potency, dosage, and delivery.

Psilocybin
4-phosphoryloxy-N, N-dimethyltryptamine

Mainly found in tropical environments, there are 144 strains of hallucinogenic Psilocybin mushrooms, with over fifty found in Mexico and over fifty more found throughout Latin America and the Caribbean.

In Mesoamerica it is believed that the mushroom was used ceremonially for millennia. The Aztecs had also used a substance called Teonanácatl or "flesh of the gods" that was believed to be Psilocybin mushrooms. Archaeologists have found that the ritual use of psychedelic mushrooms is far-reaching, explicitly represented in rock paintings dating back 9,000 years in the Sahara Desert.

Psilocybin was introduced to Westerners in the 1950's by mycologist R. Gordon Wasson who had visited Mexico in search of a "magic" mushroom, ultimately observing and partaking in rituals with the local natives. His experiences were published in Life magazine in 1957 titled, "Seeking the Magic Mushroom."

In a scientific study, it was discovered that Psilocybin successfully lifted the severe depression of all of the study's participants who had been suffering from long-term depression that anti-depressant medication could not treat. Psilocybin has also been found to alleviate and cure addiction and Post-Traumatic Stress Disorder (PTSD) and is used in therapeutic settings to alleviate the fear of death in the terminally ill.

Effects can last from 2-8 hours depending on strain, potency, dosage, and delivery.

Salvia
Salvia divinorum

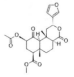

Salvia divinorum, also known as Sage of the Diviners, is a perennial herb indigenous to the Sierra Mazateca region of Oaxaca, Mexico. It is used ceremonially and touted for its medicinal healing properties by the Mazatec people to alleviate ailments such as anemia, cluster headaches, and diarrhea. In larger doses, Salvia can induce altered states of consciousness.

The first recorded mention of Salvia in Western culture was made by Jean Basset Johnson during his studies of Mazatec shamanism in the late 1930's where he had heard that they were drinking a brew made from a visionary tea. In 1962, Albert Hofmann and R. Gordon Wasson obtained a specimen from the Mazatecs, in which they described it as a "less desirable substitute" for Psilocybin.

Modern medicine has discovered its therapeutic properties and believes its active compounds may be used to treat opioid addiction, schizophrenia, chronic pain, and Alzheimer's disease. Salvia has also been proven to curb cravings for heroin and cocaine. Salvia, whose psychoactive component is *Salvinorin A*, can be consumed by smoking or vaporizing its dried leaves, but its effects tend to be shorter when smoked. Conversely, chewing its leaves tends to have longer lasting effects. There are significant variations in its psychoactivity based on a variety of phsyiological and consumption factors.

Effects can last 5-120 minutes depending on potency, dosage, and delivery.

To submit your own experience to be
considered for future volumes please visit
THE-PSYCHEDELIC-ANTHOLOGY.COM